This "diseases" by Dr. Clarke is the 6th in this collection, "Great Books in Homeopathy", designed to cheapen access to this fine art and this consistent science.

Questions, suggestions and improvements can be sent to emiliojoselemosdelima@gmail.com

Clinical questions will be submitted to our discussion group.

Good reading!

Clarke´s biography by Sue Young

John Henry Clarke 1853 – 1931

John Henry Clarke 1853–1931 was a British orthodox physician who converted to homeopathy (in ?1878 John Henry Clarke, *Homeopathy Explained*, (originally printed 1905, reprinted by Nanopathy, 1 Jan 2001). Page 5) to become a consultant at the London Homeopathic Hospitaland the editor of *The Homeopathic World* for twenty nine years.

John Henry Clarke was also the publisher of *The British Guardian,* and he was the Chairman and Vice President of *The Britons.* John Henry Clarke was called upon to give evidence in the Pemberton Billing court case in 1918 (*see below).

John Henry Clarke also met regularly with James Compton Burnett and Robert Thomas Cooper, Thomas Skinner, and others at The Cooper Club (http://www.homeoint.org/morrell/articles/pm_coope.htm See also http://homeoint.org/morrell/british/late19.htm).

John Henry Clarke wrote *Odium medicum and homeopathy*, and Edmund Becket Lord Grimthorpe wrote to *The Times* in 1888 to protest against the prejudice of the allopathic physicians in dismissing Kenneth William Millican, which resulted in a month long battle of words in *The Times.* At the close of this controversy on 20th January 1888, *The London*

Times wrote '... *So great has been the interest excited by the correspondence, that the editor has been unable to publish only a fraction of the letters sent him. The original contention was that an Odium Medicum exists, exactly analogous to the Odium Theologicum of a less enlightened age, and no less capable of blinding men...* (Federal Vanderburgh et al (Eds), *Pamphlets – homeopathic, Volume 17,* (1844 [onwards]). Page 30)'. John Henry Clarke was a student of Edward William Berridge, and he taught many lay homeopaths, including J Ellis Barker, Ephraim Connor, Edward W Cotter, John DaMonte, Thomas Maughan, Noel Puddephatt, Phyllis M Speight, Edwin D W Tomkins, Canon Roland Upcher, Frank Parker Wood, and he was a colleague of Edward Bach, Marjorie Blackie, James Compton Burnett, Robert Thomas Cooper, James Douglas Kenyon, Percival George Quinton, Thomas Skinner, John Weir, Charles Edwin Wheeler, and many others. As a teacher at the London

Homeopathic Hospital, Clarke taught Marjorie Blackie.

In 1905, John Henry Clarke heavily criticised the medical homeopaths for the lack of adequate training in homeopathy and he began to train lay practitioners, and to raise funds for a Professorship in Homeopathic Therapeutics in memory of James Compton Burnett. The British Homeopathic Association set out to meet the challenge of John Henry Clarke's criticisms. John Henry Clarke dedicated his book *Homeopathy Explained* to the British Homeopathic Association,

John Henry Clarke attended (Anon, *The Homeopathic World, Volume 43*, (1908). Page 236) the 2nd International Homeopathic Congress held in London (Anon, *The Medical Counselor, Volume 7*, (The Michigan State Homeopathic Society, 1883). Page 347) in on 11th-18th July 1881 (Anon, The Homeopathic World, (August 1,1881)) at Aberdeen House, Argyll Street, Regent Street. John Henry Clarke was a permanent secretary of the Liga Medicorum Homeopathica

Internationalis (Anon, *New England Medical Gazette, Volume 46, (1911). Page 1038).*

From Peter Morrell, British homeopathy during two centuries. (Staffordshire University, 1999). At the turn of the century there were four distinct though entangled threads emerging in UK homeopathy. They were the Cooper Club, the increased use of nosodes, the influence of James Tyler Kent and the general decline of medically qualified practice, which coincided with the rise of the lay practitioner... The second main phase of British homeopathy was undoubtedly the main figures of the Cooper Club... four distinguished homeopathic doctors used to meet regularly and were to have a major influence on its future.

These were Thomas Skinner, Robert Thomas Cooper, James Compton Burnett and John Henry Clarke... They met and dined weekly and shared their notes and experiences over a period roughly from 1880 to 1900... This group also continued to meet after the deaths of Robert Thomas Cooper and James Compton Burnett.

And, after the death of Thomas Skinner in 1906, John Henry Clarke continued the tradition by maintaining vigorous links with other major British homeopaths and by having regular meetings for the discussion of new ideas and of cases.

These meetings continuing after 1906 were with a select band of people who were in effect tutored by John Henry Clarke in all aspects of homeopathy. This also took place outside the British Homeopathic Society, with which John Henry Clarke more or less severed all contact after 1908. It also included several people who were medically unqualified amateur practitioners.

This group included Noel Puddephatt, Canon Roland Upcher and J Ellis Barker, who, as proteges of John Henry Clarke, soon became important torch bearers for the movement well into the twentieth century... I have not yet seen any material evidence that the other members of the Cooper Club taught non-doctors, but they may well have done so in secret.

It would not be surprising considering that John Henry Clarke despised the rest of his profession as traitors of homeopathy in general and of British working people in particular.

John Weir and Charles Edwin Wheeler were also members. One suspects that Edward Bach, James Douglas Kenyon, Percival George Quinton and several others were also members, and taught lay persons, though there is no direct evidence and an air of secrecy shrouds the group. The Club continued to meet into the 1930s under John Henry Clarke and Charles Edwin Wheeler...

Several key features of these doctors need emphasising. They were fiercely opposed to orthodox medical practice and made a point of castigating that system at every opportunity. Not only did they castigate it, but for the usual reasons of using suppressive, dangerous drugs which did not treat the whole person and which were unsafe and productive of only illusory change in shifting symptom patterns rather than true cure. These are the same reasons that all homeopaths have used to criticise allopathy, even from Samuel Hahnemann's day.

These blistering attacks upon orthodoxy were mainly delivered by James Compton Burnett and John Henry Clarke and usually poured forth from the pages of *The Homeopathic World*, which they edited between them at various times between 1870 and 1931. It is as if they took their cue from Samuel Hahnemann himself and so felt duty bound to 'show their mettle' by continuing a sabre rattling tradition of such attacks. As it was, the two 'camps' became utterly battle hardened and staunchly opposed, as they have remained throughout most of this century.

John Henry Clarke was a busy practitioner. As a physician he not only had his own clinic in Piccadilly, London, but he also was a consultant at the London Homeopathic Hospital and researched into new remedies — nosodes.

From *How I became a homeopath*, John Henry Clarke wrote:

"Perhaps it may not be uninteresting to reader if I state at the outset of how my own conversion to homeopathy came about. As is usually the case, I knew nothing whatsoever about homeopathy when I took a degree in surgery, since it is rarely mentioned by professors in the ordinary medical school, and then only to be misrepresented.

After my graduation as a western medical doctor at Edinburgh Medical School, by the advise of the late Angus Macdonald (one of the best friends I ever had), I took a voyage to New Zealand in charge of emigrants.

On my return, having fixed on Liverpool as a likely field in which to start practice, I asked Angus Macdonald to introduce me to some of leading doctors in that city. This he promised to do, and eventually he did – I have the letter to this day.

They were never presented, for the reasons which will be appreciated. The relatives with whom I was staying happens to be a homeopath, and they suggested that I might do worse then to go to Homeopathic Dispensary at Hardman Street, Liverpool and see what was being done there.

As the letter came not, by way of utilizing my time I went. Like Caesar, I not only 'went', but I 'saw', " but here the parallel ended – I did not conquer; instead homeopathy conquered me!

I may say that at this period, having absorbed over 80% (if marks go for anything) of the drug lore Sir Robert Christian had to impart, and having had sufficient opportunity for testing its value in practice, I had come pretty near the conclusion of Oliver Wendell Holmes saying, "If all drugs were cast into the sea, it would be so much better for man and so much the worst for the fish."

I believed then (and belief has become rather fashionable since) that the chief function of a medical man was to find out what was the matter with people – if he could; and supply them with common sense – if he happened to posses any. With duty to treat people; to cure them was out of question; and *it would be the better for honesty if he made no pretense to it.*

After few weeks of observation at the Liverpool Homeopathic Dispensary, a case was presented to me in private. A small boy of five, a relative of my own, was brought to me by his mother. Two years before, he had been badly scratched on the forehead by a cat, and when the scratches healed, a crops of warts appeared on the site of them, and there they remained up to that time in spite of different treatment by allopathic doctor.
As an allopath I could do no more than he, so I turned to homeopathy to see if that could help me. I consulted the authorities, and found that the principal drug which is credited to producing crops of warts is Thuja Occidentalis.
I ordered this, more by way of experiment than expecting much result; but I said, if there was truth in homeopathy, it ought to cure. In a few days improvement was manifest; in three weeks the warts were al gone. Rightly or wrongly I attributed, and still attribute the result to Thuja, through it

will no doubt be said that charms have done the same way.

Very well, I'd say one will give me a system of charms that I can use with precision and produce with such definite effects, I shall be very glad to try it. As it was, I concluded that if homeopathy could give me results like that, homeopathy was the system for me.

Yours faithfully
Dr J.H. Clarke, Liverpool, England.
From http://www.homeoint.org/morrell/articles/pm_clark.htm Regarding John Henry Clarke by Peter Morell. *John Henry Clarke... established himself as a very successful and highly influential London homeopath in the 1870s. But he 'fell out' with figures like Richard Hughes and Robert Ellis Dudgeon, who controlled the movement, to such an extent that all offices became closed to him, except the editorship of* The Homeopathic World, *which he retained to the end.*

He left the British Homeopathic Society in disgust, c1900, never to 'return to the fold.' He thus became a

powerful 'loose cannon' and effectively divided the movement.
This was so for two main reasons.

Firstly, he was wholly disenchanted with the direction English homeopathy had taken. He disliked the way it eventually failed to continue challenging allopathy or winning many new converts to its dwindling ranks – especially after 1900.

And it seemed to lack the will for a good fight. It simply 'gave up' in his view and came to occupy an all too cosy niche within Victorian society, conveniently devoting itself to serving solely the rich upper classes.

The second point is connected to the first: he started to teach laypersons all about homeopathy [e.g. Canon Roland Upcher, Noel Puddephatt and J Ellis Barker], towards whom many of his books were directed, and he became increasingly convinced that its future lay with them rather than with servile doctors who had 'sold out' to allopathy.

This very radical viewpoint turned out to be an astonishingly accurate premonition, really, as subsequent history has shown.

Single handedly, by the 1920s, John Henry Clarke had created a completely divided movement, composed of doctors on the one hand, and lay practitioners on the other. And it was mainly the latter who carried British homeopathy forward throughout the dismal 1930s, 40s and 50s, their light never dimming.

Yet the two strands had little contact with, and only contempt for, each other. Even in the 1960s, homeopathy was still very much a ridiculed medical minority and deep in the doldrums.

Not until the late 70s did it start taking off again, and that was mainly due to the lay revival, not to any action on the part of the doctor homeopaths – who, in fact, never lifted a finger to promote homeopathy.

And why should they? From their lucrative London practices in Harley Street and Wimpole Street?

It is quite true that Clarke was a typical early century right wing fascist and an anti Semite, which does not endear him to anyone today. How weird, therefore, that he formed such a fruitful allegiance with J Ellis Barker, who was a (radical Marxist) left winger?

J Ellis Barker was handed the editorship of The Homeopathic World *in the spring of 1932, just after John Henry Clarke died, and this brilliantly stage managed act caused great ripples of embarrassment to flow through UK homeopathy; a pervasive horror, really, that this prestigious position hadn't been passed, as expected, to another doctor, but to a lay practitioner and a German immigrant to boot!*

How sweet John Henry Clarke's revenge must have been, even from the grave! He must have lain smiling in his coffin. With some justification, John Henry Clarke regarded his fellow doctor homeopaths as the vilest of traitors to homeopathy, who had succeeded only in turning themselves into the easily manipulated and servile puppets of their rich aristocratic clientele.

He regarded them with enormous contempt.

Thus we can justly regard John Henry Clarke as the single most important English homeopath of this century and truly the darling of the movement. In terms of bold and experimental ideas and methods; for his writings; for his fierce independence; his great energy, which he poured into homeopathy with abandon; as a political force within the movement; and finally for his deep radicalism regarding lay practice, he towers like a colossus over all the rest.

From him flows nearly every tradition or strand within the fabric of modern British homeopathy, other than Kentianism.
Yet it is surely a very rich irony, that a right wing fascistshould come to be the one who turned his back on the

stuffy homeopathic establishment, accusing them of humbug in their failure to give homeopathy to the masses!

Ironic also that it took his alliance with the Marxist, J Ellis Barker, to establish a new lineage of British homeopathy, wholly devoid of any roots within the class system, and thus to truly transform it into a 'tool of liberation' Ivan Illich style....

Whatever else we might think of him as a human being, if it weren't for the wayward John Henry Clarke, and the laypersons he taught, there would be precious little homeopathy practiced in the UK today; it would still be the exclusive and minority preserve of the stuffy old rich and titled.

It was John Henry Clarke who broke the mold and it was his lay practitioners who have revived its fortunes in recent years.

Harold Fergie Woods wrote John Henry Clarke's obituary in *The Homeopathic World***, January 1932:**

From http://www.homeoint.org/biograph /clarkeen.htm '... Anyone who had met

Clarke but a few times, even only once, must have been impressed with the feeling of an exceptional human being, a forceful personality, a man apart.

He was literally a man apart, as he took his work and his mission so seriously that he gave himself very little time to mix with others. Perhaps, also, there were very few with whom he felt in harmony.

He was a prodigious worker, as his published works testify, to say nothing of the hosts of private patients from all parts of the world. He was editor of **The Homeopathic World** for altogether twenty nine years.

He was indeed an outstanding character, and if one can compare him with another, it is with him who was probably the greatest homeopath that the United States has produced James Tyler Kent.

They had the same forcible way of expressing themselves combined with an inherent retiring nature, the same intolerance of anything second rate, especially as relating to their beloved *system of therapeutics, the same scorn and contempt for time servers.*

And each gave to the world of Homeopathy the greatest and most valuable book that their respective countries have produced, indeed, in our opinion, the two most indispensable works written since the days of Samuel Hahnemann – the Dictionary of Materia Medica *and the* Repertory of Materia Medica.

John Henry Clarke wrote:

The Prescriber: How to Practise Homeopathy,
The Prescriber: A Dictionary of the New Therapeutics,
A Dictionary of Practical Materia Medica,
A Clinical Repertory to the Dictionary of Materia Medica,
Constitutional Medicine,
Vital Economy: Or, How to Conserve Your Strength,
The Enthusiasm of Homoeopathy,
Indigestion: Its Causes and Cure, Life and Work of James Compton Burnett,

The Revolution in Medicine: Being the Seventh Hahnemannian Oration Delivered ...,
What Do You Know about Homoeopathy?,
A bird's eye view of Hahnemann's Organon of medicine,
Non-surgical Treatment of Diseases of the Glands and Bones,
Radium as an Internal Remedy,
Haemorrhoids and Habitual Constipation,
Cholera, Diarrhœa, and Dysentery: Homœopathic Prevention and Cure,
Appendicitis from a homeopathic physician's point of view,
Iodide of arsenic in organic disease of the heart,
The Cure of Tumours by Medicines: With Especial Reference to the Cancer Nosodes,
Whooping-cough Cured with Pertussin, Its Homoeopathic Nosode,
Whooping-cough Cured with Coqueluchin, Its Homoeopathic Nosode,
Diseases of the Heart and Arteries,
Heart Repertory,
Catarrh, Colds and Grippe,

Cold-catching: Cold-preventing, Cold-curing, with a Section on Influenza, Rheumatism & Sciatica,
Therapeutics of the serpent poisons,
A Dictionary of Domestic Medicine,
M. Pasteur at Bay: Failure of the Experiment, M. Pasteur and Hydrophobia,
Dr. Lautaud's New Work,
The Pasteur Craze,
Homeopathy Explained,
Internal Or Homeopathic Vaccination,
Experimental Pathology Explained and Exemplified,
Gunpowder as a War Remedy,
"Physiological Cruelty".: A Reply to "Philantropos",
Our Meanest Crime (vivisection), Monkeys' Brains Once More: Schaefer V. Ferrier (vivisection),
Why the Vivisection Act is Objected to,
Odium Medicum and Homœopathy: 'The Times' Correspondence, Hahnemann and Paracelsus,
From Copernicus to William Blake,
The God of Shelley and Blake,
William Blake (1757-1827) on the Lord's Prayer,
The Call of the Sword,

What is Man?,
England Under the Heel of the Jew, a Tale of Two Books,
White Labour Versus Red, White Labour: Or, the Jew and International Politics.

CHAPTER 1 CAUSES AND CLASSIFICATION.[Causes and Classification]
DISEASES OF HEART AND ARTERIES

BY CLARKE J.H

THERE are three main divisions into which organic affections of the heart and vessels may be classed: (I,) Acute inflammatory diseases; (2,) Chronic consequences of acute inflammations; and (3,) Affections which are chronic from the beginning. To these must be added: The effects of sudden heart strain, or sudden emotions; effects of prolonged muscular over-exertion, as in athletes; faulty dress; drugging (including the effects of alcohol and tobacco); chronic kidney disease; debilitating habits; residences at high altitudes; and surgical interference with constitutional diseases.

Of all the causes which give rise to acute diseases of the heart, rheumatic fever is the most common; whooping cough, and the specific fevers (scarlatina, measles, typhoid, typhus, diphtheria, etc.), coming next in frequency. And it must not be forgotten that the heart may become the seat of inflammation primarily, from a chill, independently of any others disease, just as there may be inflammation of the lungs or any other organ from the same cause.

The serous membrane which covers the heart (pericardium), and that which lines it (endocardium) are peculiarly liable to become inflamed when the blood is charged with irritating poisons. These inflammations, as I shall show, are capable of subsiding without leaving behind any discoverable trace of their ever having occurred. Very frequently, however, permanent changes remain, which give rise to the class of heart affections which I have put second in the list.

The consequences of acute affections which remain behind are of various kinds, according to the part which was originally affected. If it was the outer covering, the result will be adherent pericardium, adhesion, that is, of the outer covering of the heart to the wall of the sac in which it moves. Strange to say this adhesion may exist to an extreme degree without giving rise to any symptoms whatever, as has been proved by post-mortem examination; the pericardium has been found to be completely adherent in patients who have not manifested the slightest sign of it during life.

The inner lining of the heart (endocardium) is a much more complicated affair than the outer covering, and consequently is much more liable to be injured by disease, and when injured to leave permanent consequences. The valves of the heart are composed of folds of the endocardium, which open and close with the heart's beat, to admit the blood to the various cavities and prevent its return.

When these valves are inflamed they do not perform their functions properly; they open too little, and so obstruct the blood's passage, or they do not close perfectly and allow the blood to escape backwards, or they do both. When inflammation subsides, the obstruction may be removed and the blood-current go on perfectly as before; or, it may not. Then, in listening over the heart, the murmuring or blowing sounds which are heard replacing some part of the normal "lupp-dupp" of the heart's beat, during the acute attack, persist afterwards. The patient finds himself short of breath on very slight exertion, and liable to palpitation of the heart and attacks of pain and faintness.

If there were not some power of compensating the disadvantage, the patient would have a miserable existence, which would soon end in death. But happily the heart is capable of a large development of strength to meet the needs of the case, "compensatory hypertrophy" occurs, and the balance is more or less completely restored; in many cases so complete is the recovery that life is not shortened, nor is its usefulness impaired.

These same membranous structures are frequently the seat of degenerative changes, independently of any permanent inflammation. The result is the same in both instances-crippling of the valves, obstruction to the blood flow, and if recovery takes place, increase in the size and strength of the heart to restore the balance.

But not only may the valves and membranes of the heart become inflamed, the muscular tissue of the heart itself may be weakened and degenerated, and also the vessels which supply it with blood. In all these cases there is present some chronic poison in the organism-most probably one or other (or a combination) of the three chronic "miasms" of Hahnemann-Psora, syphilis, or sycosis.

In this connection I may refer to one of the other causes which I have mentioned as being responsible for many cases of heart disease, namely, surgical interference with constitutional affections. In my work on "Non-Surgical Treatment of Diseases of the Glands and Bones," I have instanced a case in which the removal of diseased glands was followed by the onset of disease of the aortic valve of the heart. Another fruitful cause of it is to be found in operations for piles. A painful instance of this came under my own notice, which I will now relate.

CASE I.-AORTIC VALVULAR DISEASE CONSEQUENT ON OPERATION FOR PILES. FATAL ENDING.

Sir S.E., a prominent Indian civilian, consulted me some years ago about a persistent cold in the head.

Enquiring into its origin I found it had continued for about two years, dating from a time a little subsequent to an operation he had undergone for piles. The piles gave him but little inconvenience, but he was persuaded to have them "cured" by operation. Of course an operation never did, and never could "cure" piles : it can only remove the haemorrhoidal swellings, without touching the constitutional condition on which they depend. The constitutional disease from which Sir S.E. suffered would be called "Psora" by Hahnemann, and "Gout" by other pathologists. The basis of gout (as I hope at some future time to show) is the psoric miasm of Hahnemann. Be that as it may, the operation was performed; the cold in the head came on-and something much worse than that. Noticing a peculiar quality in the patient's pulse, I made a cursory examination of his heart, and there found extensive degeneration of the aortic valve. On my putting one or two questions, but in such a way as not to excite any alarm, my patient said he knew his heart was all right, "The doctors examined me carefully and said it was quite sound before I was put under the anesthetic." Beyond giving general directions I said no more about it, as it could not have helped matters to have done so; but the sequence of events was quite clear to me. Before the operation he had no heart disease.

The operation disturbed the morbid constitutional element, which at that time had a practically safe and innocent expression in the piles, and sent it in upon more vital parts of the organism. The chronic nasal catarrh and the diseased heart were the consequences. Sir S.E. only called upon me twice. A few months later I read in The Times that he had been found dead in his bed at an hotel in Edinburgh. I have no hesitation in saying that to operate for piles is as dangerous as it is unnecessary. Piles are not by any means difficult to cure by constitutional means, and when cured thus the patient is cured, and no dangerous after- effects are to be feared.

Among other causes of heart disease I have mentioned sudden emotions. The popular expression "Died of a broken heart" is not altogether figurative. It is possible for the heart to rupture from great emotion, but I am inclined to think the heart that does rupture under these conditions could not have been thoroughly sound to begin with. The majority of cases of "broken heart" are due to aneurism within the pericardium. But short of rupture, cases of dilatation of the heart do occur from strong emotion. Here is a case in point, which exemplifies the action of Iodide of arsenic. **CASE II.-DILATATION OF THE RIGHT SIDE OF THE HEART AND THINNING OF ALL ITS WALLS, DUE TO SUPPRESSED EMOTION. RELIEF FROM Iodide of Arsenic AND OTHER REMEDIES.**

The patient was a lady age. 68, who came under my care in July, 1881. Her illness dated from five years before. She has lived in the West Indies and has had much trouble. The first indication of heart disease she traced to suppressed emotion; she felt as if her heart would burst, but endured it and said nothing; she had frequent fits of dyspnoea on exertion and fits of "asthma," which were relieved if she took wine. Afterwards she had frequent attacks of bronchitis, which made matters worse. When I saw her first she complained of breathlessness on the least exertion, a stoppage when she lay on the left side, but no pain. The feet were cold but did not swell. As long as she kept quite quiet and warm she was fairly comfortable. I found evidence of slight chronic bronchial irritation, and the examination of the heart showed the following condition :- Area of dullness increased. Apex beat not felt. No tenderness. No bruit. No reduplication. Second sound slightly accentuated in pulmonary area. The sounds are weak but regular for some time; then they become irregular and fluttering for a few beats. Sometimes there was a flutter and a stop. I never could detect anything wrong with the valves.

There was dilatation of the right side, displacing the apex, feebleness of action making no perceptible impression on the chest walls, indicating degeneration rather than hypertrophy. She received benefit from Arsenic 3, and Digit.1. Some months afterwards she had an attack of bronchitis, and I put her on the Iodide with Bry. after Hepar and Kali bichrom. had done some good. The improvement became more rapid, and soon she was what she considered well. The following year in another attack I again treated her with the Iodide with the same result-improvement both of the heart and lung symptoms. She said the Iodide seemed to "soothe her to sleep." In the early part of 1883 she had another attack. She was then out of the reach of homoeopathy, and she did not recover. I heard that she died quite quietly and painlessly.

CHAPTER 2 CURABILITY OF VALVULAR DISEASE OF THE HEART IN THE ACUTE STAGE. [Curability Of Valvular Disease] As I have stated before, it is not to be expected that old-established valvular disease should be altered, or destroyed valves restored, though even in these cases much may be done by remedies to restore the power of the heart when it is defective, and to bring about proper compensation, which is practically a cure. In recent cases of valve affection, on the other hand, it has frequently been my lot to observe the disappearance of all signs of disease under treatment. In my book on "Rheumatism" I have mentioned, among others, a case of this kind which particularly struck me when I was resident medical officer at the London Homoeopathic Hospital. It was that of a young girl who had a severe attack of acute rheumatism, with both pericarditis and endocarditis. Under treatment, the friction sounds of the pericardial inflammation quite disappeared, and when these had gone the bruits indicating endocardial mischief also subsided.

One of the chief difficulties in the treatment of endocarditis occurring in connection with rheumatic fever lies in the fact that there are so few symptoms indicating the mischief.

Pericarditis has generally abundance of symptoms, hence it is a much easier matter to cure cases of this. On the other hand, there may be very extensive endocarditis and no sign be given except on physical examination. In such cases the only thing to be done is to take the totality of the symptoms and to prescribe accordingly. If there are no symptoms elsewhere to guide, such medicines as have been found in practice or in provings to have an affinity for the lining membrane of the heart and arteries should be thought of, when the constitution of the patient and his previous medical history, with any former symptoms he may have had, will serve to distinguish the most similar.

The two valves of the heart which are most liable to inflammation are the mitral, which transmits the blood from the left auricle to the left ventricle of the heart; and the aortic, through which the contraction (or "beat" of the heart) propels the blood from the left ventricle into the arteries of the body. Any narrowing of these valves obstructs the flow of the blood, and any defect in their closure allows the blood to pass backwards through them. These defects give rise to certain abnormal sounds called bruits, or murmurs, which take the place of the proper sounds produced by the valves. The normal sound of the heart is a double sound which has been fairly represented by the syllables "lupp-dupp," the first part of it occurring when the ventricles of the heart contract (systole), and the second when they open again (diastole).

The auricles which receive the blood- the right from the body, the left from the lungs-contract just before the ventricles, but as they have much less arduous work to do they are much less powerful than the ventricles, and normally their action is unaccompanied by any sound. When, however, these valves are narrowed (that of the right ventricle is called the tricuspid, that of the left the mitral), a murmur is heard over the area of the valve just before the heart beats, and is hence called pre- systolic. When the mitral valve is defective it does not close perfectly; when the heart beats the blood is driven back into the left auricle and causes a systolic murmur instead of a click. This explains the breathlessness that accompanies many forms of heart disease, for the pressure is thrown back on the blood- vessels of the lungs and the blood is not properly aerated. Thus a pre-systolic murmur heard over the area of the mitral valve (that is, roughly, over the point where the heart is felt beating) denotes obstruction to the flow, and a systolic murmur heard in the same area denotes regurgitation. The area at which aortic sounds are best heard is at the spot where the second left rib joins on to the breast bone. The opening of the aortic valve occurs at the time of the heart's beat (systole or first sound) and then any narrowing of its orifice causes a systolic murmur.

If it does not close perfectly at the time of the second syllable of the "lupp-dupp" a murmur is heard and is called diastolic. When it is both narrowed and does not close perfectly a double murmur is heard, something like a sawing sound, replacing the proper sounds altogether.

The other two valves, which are much

less frequently affected, are the tricuspid and the pulmonary. The tricuspid transmits the blood from the right auricle (which receives it after it has circulated through the body) to the right ventricle; and the pulmonary valve (which is in the pulmonary artery) transmits the blood, when the ventricles contract, from the right ventricle into the lungs. The sounds of the tricuspid valve are best heard on the level of the fourth rib close to the left edge of the sternum or breast bone (or, if the ventricle is enlarged, on the right edge of the sternum at the same level); the pulmonary area is in the interspace between the first and second ribs, close to the left edge of the sternum.

Sounds of blood regurgitating into the left auricle when the mitral valve is defective are often best heard just to the left and a little below the pulmonary area, where a part of the left auricle approaches the surface.

There are many other variations from the normal in the quality of the "lupp-dupp" besides the occurrence of murmurs, each indicating some particular condition of the heart. For instance, if the two sides of the heart do not act absolutely synchronously either or both of the sounds may be reduplicated. On the other hand, the presence of a murmur is not an absolute sign of valve defects. It may be brought about by other causes such as the condition of the blood.

The size of the heart is estimated by the size of the area which gives a dull sound when percussion is made on the front of the chest.

The sphygmographic tracings (which show the rapidity of the heart's beats and all the vibrations the wall of the artery goes through between one beat and the next) are all taken with Dr. Dudgeon's pocket Sphygmograph (pulse-writer) which has superseded every other. Dr. Dudgeon has explained the instrument in an exceedingly interesting little work entitled "The Sphygmograph," and published by Balliere, Tindall & Cox.

During the summer of 1892 a numbers of cases of endocarditis came under my observation in connection with acute fevers. There was at the time an extensive epidemic of German measles and the first case I shall describe is that of a young lady aged 19, who was one of its victims.

CASE III.-INFLAMMATION OF THE MITRAL VALVE OF THE HEART IN A CASE OF GERMAN MEASLES. RECOVERY UNDER TREATMENT.

On June 15, 1892, I called to see Miss L., who had been somewhat ill for four days. I found the rash of German measles, sore throat, the right tonsil being enlarged. There was a cough, and she raised a good deal of phlegm. There was some fever. The monthly period was on at the time. The pulse was 72. On listening to the heart I found a systolic mitral bruit. She had cold clammy feet. Under Belladonna 30 the symptoms of the fever left her, but the bruit remained. On the 22nd of June the bruit was audible in the mitral, tricuspid and left auricular areas when she was lying down, but disappeared when she sat up. There was slight giddiness when walking and she was tired of sitting up. I gave her Spigelia 30, and in a few days the bruit became less distinct. She afterwards received Nat. mur. and then Arsen. for other indications; but on June 29th, after a restless night, hot and perspiring, the pulse was 84, the mitral bruit was very distinct, and heard in all the areas of the heart, and the patient felt "queer," so I again gave Spigelia 30. Two days after this I found her feeling much better, and I could not hear the bruit. A few days later I listened again, but could hear nothing of it, so I let her leave town for the seaside.

CASE IV.—ACUTE INFLAMMATION OF MITRAL VALVE ACCOMPANYING GERMAN MEASLES AND MENTAL STRAIN. RECOVERY.

About the same time I was attending another German measles patient, also a young lady, who developed in the course of it a similar affection of the mitral valve. Eventually this also disappeared, but as this case was more complicated, the attack having supervened on a long period of overwork and mental strain, much longer time was required. The medicine which had most effect on the heart symptoms in this case was Baryta carb., which was given in two-grain doses of the 3x. The sensations she complained of were a strained feeling referred to the base of the heart and a sharp pain about the apex. The 3x appeared to have more decided action in this case than the 30th which was given first.

CASE V.—ENDOCARDITIS OCCURRING IN MEASLES. PARTIAL DISAPPEARANCE OF MURMUR; COMPLETE COMPENSATION.

Charlie W., aged 10, had an attack of English measles in May, 1892. I saw him on the 28th, and all the classical symptoms of the disease were present, and, in addition, a mitral systolic bruit. There were no symptoms arising from the latter and I treated the case according to the symptoms in the ordinary way.

Under Bell. 30, Merc. sol.30, and

Sulph.30, the disease ran a mild course, leaving the boy well, except for the bruit. On May 7th, as there were no symptoms, I put him on Lycopus virginicus 1x, which has a reputation in valvular disease. I could trace no effect to this, nor to Spongia 30, with which I followed it. On 17th of May, taking into consideration that he came of a consumptive family on one side of the house, and guided by the crenated appearance of his teeth, which Dr. Burnett has shown is an indication for the medicine, I gave one dose of Bacillinum 200, and as he had cold, clammy feet, I followed this with Calc. carb. Under this treatment he made good progress, and on the 10th of June I ceased attending. The bruit was then inaudible when he stood up but could be heard if he lay down.

On December 14th I saw him again for something else, and had the opportunity of examining the heart. He told me he had no shortness of breath on running up stairs, and he could run as well as ever he could. The apex beat was felt in the fifth space, further to the left than normal, and the area of cardiac dullness was greater than normal. On standing no bruit was audible; there was a little accentuation of the first sound at the apex and of the second over the pulmonary artery. On making him lie down I found that the bruit reappeared in all the areas, loudest over the apex, and the action of the heart became irregular.

I have not been able satisfactorily to account to myself for this condition in which there is competence of the valve in the erect, and incompetence in the recumbent position, but it is a condition I have often observed. In one case, that of a child who had at one time unmistakable incompetence of the mitral valve with attacks of violent palpitation and flushing of eyes and face following whooping-cough, I found, after some years, that the bruit could only be heard when she lay down; and still later it could not be heard at all. There was no anaemia in this case. Some defect of the posterior flap of the valve, or irregular action of the columnae cardiae may possibly account for it.

I will now relate another case of very extensive heart inflammation which resulted in a practical cure. CASE VI.-ACUTE INFLAMMATION OF THE PERICARDIUM AND VALVES OF THE HEART. PROMPT ACTION OF Spigelia. RECOVERY.

On the 22nd June, 1889, James T., a chimney-sweep, aged 44, came to my hospital clinic on the recommendation of a private patient of mine who had persuaded him to try Homoeopathy. When he entered my out-patients' room it was easy to see he was exceedingly ill.

Like most of his class he had led a hard, reckless life. He commenced chimney-sweeping as a tiny boy in the days when boys were sent up the flues instead of the machine brushes now used. Naturally he was a man of powerful physique; but now it had been with the greatest difficulty that he had succeeded in reaching the hospital. He had the blurred, heavy look of countenance-a sort of indistinctness of features-sometimes noticed in sufferers from heart disease. He felt just as ill as he looked, for he afterwards told me that he never expected to reach home again alive.

Fourteen days before, he had taken cold from getting wet during a trip to Oxford on the river. This was followed by a cough with raising of thick phlegm, the cough being so painful that he had to hold himself, and this had continued. The chief thing he now complained of was a pain at the heart as if it were swelling up. The pain gradually moved down, and the night before his visit to me was in the left flank; then it moved up to the heart again. Sensation as if a big knife went through it, aggravated on taking a breath. The pain prevented him from sleeping; it was impossible for him to lie on the left side. Tongue white; appetite good, but he could not eat, because eating brought on the pain. Bowels confined; he had a choking sensation in the epigastrium, and a dizziness in the eyes.

On examining the heart I found there was an increase in size, a pericardial rub, and bruits in the aortic and mitral areas; that is to say, there was pericarditis with effusion and endocarditis as well.

The knife-like pain in the heart singled out Spigelia from all the other medicines related to his condition, so I gave it him in the third centesimal dilution, a dose every hour.

He slept well that night, as he was able to breathe better. The next day I called at his house, and I found a decrease in the pericardial rubbing sound, and a diminution in the area of cardiac dullness.

June 24th.-Still better; sleeps well; has no pain; appetite good. On this day I made the following notes of the state of the heart:-

Slight rub heard over centre of heart.

Mitral area: double bruit, the systolic

portion being heard in the axilla.

Tricuspid area (right border of sternum on level of fourth rib) : a double rough grating sound.

Aortic area: a double bruit.

On the night of the 25th-26th (as his wife informed me) his breathing seemed to be arrested; it began again with a gasp.

The Spigelia 3 was continued all this time, though it was not given so frequently as at first. From the 25th it was given every two hours.

A few weeks after this he mentioned a circumstance which occurred during the time he was taking Spigelia-the loss of a pain in the right knee which had troubled him for eighteen months. If he knelt on it he was unable to get up without going down on the other knee as well, and then stretching out the right leg. The pain was as if the knee got out of joint. He had been sometimes for hours at night before he could get it into the right position in bed. He asked me if my medicine could have had anything to do with its disappearance; for as he had not told me anything about it before, he did not see how I could have cured it. On referring to Allen, I found this in italics: Tearing pain, like a sprain, in the left knee, only when walking, so that at times he limped, since he could not bend the knee as usual. Other similar symptoms refer to the right knee and both knees. That the Spigelia must have the credit of this bye-cure I proved later on, for the pain in the knee returned; but a few doses of the Spigelia 1m F.C. permanently removed it.

But to go back. By July 1st he was quite free from any chest symptoms: he could lie on either side. But he was weak in the calves, had giddiness, and suffered from constipation with straining. Nux 1m relieved the latter condition.

On July 3rd he was still complaining of weakness in the legs, so I put him on

Baryta. c. 1m, after which there was rapid improvement.

He continued on this medicine, with a rest, till August 10th. Occasionally he had palpitation on lying down at night; on the 5th there was slight pain in lower part of left chest; on the 12th numbness of left shoulder and arm. On August 1st he had an attack of giddiness in the evening whilst walking in the street. He resumed work on the 9th of August. On October 11th he declared he felt as well as ever he did in his life. Being an enthusiastic member of the Volunteer force, he had been testing his powers by practising ball-firing. The following Easter he went through the fatigues and exposure of the Easter Volunteer manoeuvres, indulging himself even (without asking my permission, I need hardly say) in bathing in the cold spring sea.

On the 19th of March, 1893, I called upon him to make an examination of his present condition. For the last eighteen months he has been better, he says, than for years before. His pulse was 72, regular, steady and of good force. I append his sphygmogram, taken from the left radial, standing, with a pressure of 3 1/2 ounces. It does not differ from a normal tracing except, perhaps, in the strength and sharpness of the upstroke and sudden though quickly arrested return.

Examination.-The area of dullness is still greater than normal; the apex beat is felt in the sixth interspace and more to the left than normal. Coming to the heart sounds, I find, of course, no pericardial rub. Also the mitral bruit and the grating sound (probably pericardial) in the tricuspid area are no longer to be heard. The double aortic bruit still remains. In the tricuspid area the first sound is clear, and a soft bruit replaces the second. This is probably the aortic diastolic propagated downwards. In the mitral area the first sound is somewhat impure-not the clear, sharp click of a normal valve-but there is no bruit, showing that the valve is competent.

In this case I conclude that under the treatment-that is, under the action of Spigelia and Baryta carb. chiefly-the inflammation of the heart, which affected both the outer and inner lining, was subdued, and the affection of the mitral valve was so far remedied that it has been restored to competence. The aortic valves remained still as they were, but the softness of the systolic portion of the double bruit shows that the degree of obstruction to the blood-flow is but slight, and the softness of the diastolic part that the regurgitation is not considerable. This shows that there has been, at any rate, an arrest of the disease process, and I am disposed to think that the aortic trouble dates from before the time when I first saw him.

I may say that after having been a very heavy drinker, he suddenly gave up alcohol in all forms seven years before this illness began. What made him give it up was that he lost nerve when at his work on roofs, and even on stepping from a curbstone into the street felt as if he would fall. Afterwards he suffered much from "indigestion," and in the night violent palpitation and sometimes arrest of breathing, as noticed by his wife. Loss of nerve is a very common symptom in heart affections, and the probability is that the aortic disease was commencing at that time. CASE VII.-ULCERATIVE ENDOCARDITIS ENDING FATALLY, THE AUTOPSY REVEALING A HEALED PATCH ON A SPOT WHERE INFLAMMATION HAD OCCURRED DURING AN EARLIER ATTACK OF ACUTE RHEUMATISM.

Before proceeding further I would like to refer to a case of ulcerative endocarditis following pneumonia, with delirium tremens, which I published in the November number of The Homoeopathic World for 1884 (vol. xix., p. 497). The case ended fatally, but the point I wish to refer to was made evident at the post-mortem examination. The heart weighed thirteen ounces.

On the under surface of the aortic valves (which were competent) grew abundant granulations like cauliflower excrescences, exuding purulent matter. These granulations pressed against the aortic segment of the mitral valve, constricting the orifice artificially. The mitral valve itself was healthy, except that the remains of an old deposit were found between its laminae.

Now this patient (who was a groom, and, like many of his class, addicted to spirit drinking) had been in the hospital under my care some years before with a severe attack of acute rheumatism, and during the attack there were no signs of the heart being affected. But that there had been some inflammation of the valve, and that it had healed without causing deformity, this white patch found on the mitral valve at the post-mortem examination proved. In the second attack, the aortic valve was the one which was affected by the morbid process.

Here is another case in which a murmur disappeared.
CASE VIII.-ACUTE RHEUMATISM WITH HEART INVOLVEMENT.

DISAPPEARANCE OF MURMUR UNDER TREATMENT.

Walter L., aged 21, compositor, was admitted to London Homoeopathic Hospital, January 12th, 1893, having been taken ill seven days before with pains in joints of left leg.

Two days later the right leg became affected, and he took to bed. He then noticed that the slightest exertion brought on a severe pain near the upper part of the chest. He perspired a good deal. He had never had rheumatism before.

On admission, the joints of the lower limbs were painful on movement, right arm stiff, joints painful, and slightly swollen. Temperature varied from 99 degree to 100.2 degree. On the 14th when I saw him for the first time the following was the condition of the heart: Mitral bruit rather indistinct. Apex beat in fifth interspace, which is indrawn. There was a copious deposit of phosphates in the urine, but no albumen. Headache in temples; some perspiration.

There could be little doubt about the medicine in this case. All symptoms pointed to Bryonia, and I gave it in the twelfth potency, a dose every hour. For the first two days he had received Spigelia 3x, prescribed by the resident physician on account of the condition of the heart. There had been some amelioration of the chest pain, but the general condition was unchanged. Under Bryonia there was rapid subsidence of all symptoms, the chest pain more particularly. On the 25th he received Merc. viv.12, and on February 1st Sulph. 30. He left, cured, on February 3rd. On the 28th January a careful examination of the heart failed to reveal any murmur.

I will now relate two cases in which, though the valve defect was not removed, compensation occurred and a practical cure resulted. The first was a very remarkable one, as few who saw the patient at her worst expected that she would recover.

CASE IX.-ACUTE RHEUMATIC

ENDOCARDITIS. MITRAL SYSTOLIC AND PRE-SYSTOLIC BRUITS; ATTACKS OF ANGINA; CURE BY COMPENSATION; ACTION OF Crocus.

I now come to a case in which the resources of homoeopathy were markedly illustrated by the prompt effect it showed of the simillimum, given purely on symptomatic indications; the medicine, so far as I know, never having been given in a case of organic heart disease before.

Katie F., aged 19, was admitted to the Hospital on November 11th, 1893, having had two attacks of rheumatic fever previously, the second, three years before admission. Ever since this attack she had suffered off and on from attacks of breathlessness, lasting from a few minutes to over a week; the slightest exertion at any time gave rise to breathlessness. Four days before admission, she awoke in the night with severe pain over the right half of the liver anteriorly.

The pain spread up to the neck and seemed to cause shortness of breath. During the day the pain extended all over the chest, and the shortness of breath was worse. Motion made the pain worse, and also lying flat; she was obliged to be propped up during the greater part of her stay in the hospital. On the day following this seizure she was taken with pains in all her joints and neck simultaneously. At the same time a rash appeared on her forearms, which she described as consisting of little white bumps at first, these subsiding, and leaving small red rings. The rash was accompanied with itching, and disappeared in twenty-four hours. On admission, all the pains persisted, and the dyspnoea. The pulse was 126, and the temperature 99.2 degree. On two occasions during her stay in the hospital, the temperature went up to 102 degree. This was during extreme attacks of angina pectoris, and a low typhoid condition, which made me apprehend ulcerative endocarditis. During the attacks she was in imminent danger. With the exception of the occasions mentioned, the temperature oscillated between 97 degree and 99.6 degree. It was subnormal on admission. She received Baptisia 30 at first, and improved for some days. Spigelia, Lachesis 12, Mercurius vivus 12, Arsenicum 12, and Veratrum alb.3 during attacks of angina (collapse, pain, cold sweat on forehead) all gave considerable help.

The condition of the heart was as follows:-A thrill was felt over the region of the apex. A mitral systolic and pre-systolic bruit was heard over the apex, indicating constriction and incompetence of the mitral valve. The heart's action was exceedingly rapid, as much as 132 per minute. The following is a sphygmogram taken on January 23rd at a pressure of three ounces.

On February 7th the only abnormal sound to be heard was a loud pre-systolic bruit, with a thump at that end of it; at that time the pain in the chest was worse than usual-an aching under the sternum with internal soreness. On other occasions the pain extended to left shoulder, but not down the arm.

On April 12th, when she was convalescent and able to walk about, this was the condition: Thrill felt over apex area, loud systolic bruit at apex prolonged into axilla, heard also in left auricular area, and faintly in aortic.

No definite pre-systolic heard. At the foot of previous page is the sphygmogram taken two days later, also at a pressure of three ounces.

On April 15th, just before she went out, I again examined the condition of the heart :- No thrill over apex. Beat rather forcible, area tender to pressure.

Loudish systolic bruit over apex, propagated into axilla. Listening near the left edge of the sternum, a very soft pre- systolic is heard as well as the systolic.

Systolic heard in left auricular area and slightly in aortic area.

Sounds in pulmonary and tricuspid

areas fairly clear. She went on steadily improving, and when she left the hospital on April 22nd she could walk up and down stairs without difficulty.

It may be noted that as the regurgitation murmur (systolic) became more marked and the obstructive murmur (pre-systolic) less so, the patient's condition improved. In some manner the constriction of the mitral valve became less during the illness, allowing freer passages of the blood stream in both directions.

I will now tell how I came to give the patient Crocus, the medicine which gave most signal help, and materially expedited her recovery.

On February 24th, whilst I was in the ward seeing another patient, Katie F. was seized with a fit of uncontrollable laughter apropos of some trifle. I put on her tongue a dose of Crocus 30, which immediately quieted her. On March 29th, though much better, she still had a good deal of pain in the chest; on asking her to describe the pain, she said it was of a "jumping" character. Putting this, the internal jumping sensation as if of something alive, which is a characteristic of Crocus, with the old symptom of uncontrollable laughter, I was led to give her that medicine in the thirtieth potency three or four times a day. She immediately began to make rapid advance. The "jumping" steadily subsided. She was soon able to be up and eat ordinary food, and needed no other medicine till the end of the case.

Crocus has a number of heart symptoms including "stitches and shocks." But the most characteristic symptom is as if something were hopping or jumping in the chest.

CASE X.-ACUTE RHEUMATISM WITH ENDOCARDITIS AND EFFUSION INTO THE
PERICARDIUM. ACTION OF Merc. viv. COMPENSATION ESTABLISHED.

Daisy K., aged 6, admitted into the hospital in February, 1893, was first seen by me on February 4th.

She had then been ill about a week, complaining of pains in the feet. Right knee and right hand and fingers were swollen. Tongue covered with thick white fur; throat reddened but no patches; pain on swallowing. The patient was very much prostrated; she was worse at night, screaming with pain nearly all night long. There was marked increase in the area of cardiac dullness, showing effusion into the pericardium, and a mitral systolic bruit. The patient complained of pain in the region of the heart. The temperature had been up to 102 degree. There was much night perspiration.

Before I saw her she had received Aconite, Bryonia, and Belladonna, the last of which had given some relief. The patient was, however, in great distress, and the symptoms-pain and effusion into joints and pericardium, white tongue, heavy perspirations, and with marked aggravation of symptoms at night- pointed so strongly to Mercurius, that I prescribed that medicine.

Treatment Merc. viv. 12, one drop in water every hour for four doses, and then every two hours.

There was an immediate change for the better as the next day's report showed.

February 5th.-Patient had a very good night. The right side is now quite well. The left knee, ankle, and (slightly) the left hand are swollen. Temperature lower. Repeat.

February 7th.-Better; heart dullness diminished in extent; child less fretful. Repeat every four hours.

February 11th.-Temperature normal, heart dullness now normal, showing that the effusion was re-absorbed. No pain anywhere; tongue still coated. Repeat.

February 18th.-The general condition is now quite good; the systolic bruit is still present, but there are no symptoms.

On February 20th I gave Calcarea 30, leaving off the Mercurius; and on the 24th I changed the prescription to Arsen. 12. She left the hospital on March 4th perfectly well in all respects, except the defect of the mitral valve; but this was so far compensated that it gave rise to no symptoms whatever.

CHAPTER 3 REMEDIAL POWER OF HOMOEOPATHY IN CASES OF CHRONIC HEART DISEASE. [Remedial Power in Chronic Heart Disease] WHEN once the muscular fibres of the heart have become weakened, so that the organ is no longer able to discharge its functions without effort, no matter what the cause of the weakening may have been, the symptoms are very similar-breathlessness and palpitation on the slightest exertion, inability to lie down flat, or to lie on the left side, pains in the heart of many kinds, and varying in intensity from very slight to the agonies of angina pectoris. These symptoms occur in chronic cases of valve disease, in cases of fatty degeneration of the muscular fibres of the heart, in accumulation of fat about the heart when it is an accompaniment of general obesity.

I will now relate a number of cases, all more or less chronic, in which chronic affections of the heart were materially and permanently relieved by homoeopathic treatment. I will first give some of the earlier ones from the series treated with Iodide of arsenic. Some of these cases are defective as therapeutic observations in that more than one medicine was given on the same day, but in spite of this I think it is possible to determine the action of the medicines given.

CASE XI.-MITRAL STENOSIS AND INCOMPETENCE WITH ANGINA. CO-EXISTENCE OF NASAL POLYPUS. PRACTICAL CURE WITH Iodide of arsenic AND OTHER REMEDIES.

Mrs. McC, age 52, rather above medium size, grey eyes, dark hair, thin, rather pale, consulted me April 22nd, 1882. She was taken ill in Scotland the previous July. She went to bed one night quite well, and woke up with a feeling as if the ribs were being pressed into the heart; for thirty-six hours was in agony. It was a month before she was well enough to travel to London. She still has the same sensation (of pressing-in of the ribs) and palpitation at the same time. Has had two or three attacks since that in July, but not so severe or long-lasting. Has frequent severe palpitation and rush of blood; is faint after the attack. In the night she wakes with a feeling of going over a precipice. If the feeling comes on when she goes to bed she cannot sleep at all and has to be propped up. She cannot go upstairs or exert herself, as it brings on pain in the side-not the pain at the heart; that comes on when she is quite calm and still.

She has a cough night and morning and raises much phlegm. Has to be very careful with her diet. Never was strong; for ten years attended the Victoria Park Hospital for Consumption. Had her right arm broken twice, at six and at sixteen.

Since the second break has had

rheumatism in the arm, but never had rheumatic fever. On this day I had not time to examine the chest thoroughly, but I took the following sphygmogram, and told her to return in a week.

The sphygmogram taken on this day is of great interest, the beat being apparently triple. The beat, however, is not really triple. The first figure represents a natural beat. This is followed by a double beat, the secondary pulsation being so slight as not to be perceptible to the finger on the pulse. The second and subsequent sphygmograms show only double beats until, under treatment, the beats become quite normal and regular.

April 29th.-She reported that she had a very bad cold, and was coughing much; the cough being in fits. She raised a good deal of phlegm at night. Pulse 46.

I was now able to make a complete examination of the chest, with the result that the heart was found much enlarged and the valve action defective. Subsequent examination showed that it was the mitral valve which was at fault, being narrowed and incompetent. There was some anaemia, and some consolidation of the apex of the right lung. Here are the particulars of the examination on that date :-

Vertical dullness begins at lower border of third costal cartilage. Transverse dullness at level of fourth costal cartilage extends two and a half inches to the left of the sternum. This part is bulged forwards. The apex beat is felt, but very faintly; the impulse is felt near the sternum.

Sounds : regularly irregular. One strong beat is felt, followed by two smaller ones which make no impression on the pulse at the wrist. Sometimes there is a soft systolic bruit, and at the tricuspid area a rough bruit apparently diastolic. The heart-sounds are clear at pulmonary and aortic areas. Bruit de diable in neck.

Lungs: dullness and slight flattening with increased vocal resonance and fremitus at right apex exaggerated expiration.

Treatment Arsen. iod., gr. ij, night and morning after food; Digitalis I, one drop in water three times a day.

May 6th.-First part of week worse; twice she fainted right away, but last part of week much better, less fluttering, less flushing; cough looser.

Examination.-The secondary beat is felt like a thump at the apex, where a soft systolic bruit is heard with the primary beat; it is heard nowhere else. The region of the apex is very sensitive. Repeat medicines.

May 20th.-She is very much better; has not had the heart so quiet for months, only has palpitation now when called suddenly, and that only slight. Appetite good, but she cannot take meat.

Examination.-Action of the heart quiet and regular, but instead of the two sounds three are heard; after the systolic comes the diastolic and then a sort of rebound. With the systolic sound, in the mitral area and over the third left costal cartilage a soft systolic bruit is heard.

This is not heard with the third sound, and it is not heard to the right of the sternum. In the aortic area the first is very feeble and the second stronger. In the pulmonary area all three sounds are heard, but not the bruit. Repeat.

June 3rd.—Keeping very much better. Phlegm hard to raise.

Examination.—Lungs: prolonged expiration both apices and increased vocal resonance, the latter most marked on right side, with increased vocal fremitus. Heart-sounds much steadier, there is a thump with the first sound; a presystolic bruit can now be distinctly made out in mitral area; no apex beat is felt; cardiac dullness extends from half an inch to right of sternum five inches across.

Treatment Kali bich., 3; one drop to be taken occasionally when expectoration was difficult. Otherwise the same medicines to be continued.

After this I did not see the patient again for over a year. She returned on August 25th, 1883. Her condition on this date was as follows: Pulse 82, has no pain at heart now, though she feels it weak and is faint; there is a presystolic thrill.

She came now to consult me on account of blocking of the nose and loss of taste and smell. I discovered a polypus in each nostril, the right the larger. Eighteen years before she had had polypus, which she said was burnt.

Arsen. iod. 3x was given night and morning; Thuja 3x, one drop in water four times a day; Thuja 0 to be applied with brush three times a day.

September 8th.-Heart better, pulse 76. Not so faint and low. Tastes better, can smell sometimes. Sleep poor. Repeat.

September 19th.-Unable to sleep since

15th; has the "falling" sensation; continual fidgeting with the limbs. Pulse regular.

Treatment Act. r. I, one drop four times a day; Coffea 3, one drop every hour if sleepless; Thuja 0 to be applied.

October 3rd.-Very much better. Sleep good after three days; fidgetiness better; nose better-less stopped. Repeat.

October 24th.-Very much better generally, can smell now and then.

November 14th.-Very much better; smells quite well, tastes better, sleeps well. Repeat.

December 5th.-Very much better as regards the polypus, it gives no inconvenience now. Heart troublesome again; sleep not so good. Has pressure on the back of the head. The application of Thuja now causes pain.

December 29th.-In the early part of this year she had a great shock-the news of the wreck of a ship on board of which she had a son. She was for many days in suspense as to his fate, but learned at last that he was among the saved. She does not think she has been well since the shock. She has nausea after all food. Tongue white; bowels confined. Has pain in the side. Nose fairly clear. Presystolic still heard, only faintly, at apex. Pulse a little irregular; cough in fits; sleep bad till she used Coffea. Thuja still causes pain.

Treatment Arsen. iod. 3x, a grain night and morning; Ign. I, one drop four times a day; Thuja application.

January 12th, 1884.-Very much better. Had a faint on December 31st, but much better on the 2nd and has continued so. Bowels rather difficult Nose a little stopped; has flushes. Repeat.

February 23rd.-Says she is "pretty well," the polypus is the worst of her troubles. Is losing taste and smell; has rheumatism in left foot and arm.

Treatment Thuja 3x, one drop three times a day; repeat Thuja locally, and Arsen, iod. night and morning.

March 12th.-Better; nose better, tastes better, has little pain. Repeat.

April 12th.-Has neuralgia; nose pretty well, has been able to smell for the last fortnight.

Treatment Spigelia I, one drop four times a day.

This case was two years under observation. The patient came originally for an opinion merely, not expecting to receive much benefit, as she knew she had heart-disease and considered it hopeless. She was restored under treatment to activity and comfort, and I ascribe the chief share of the credit to the Iodide of arsenic.

In the case I shall now relate there will be less room for doubt as to the drug which worked the cure as the treatment was less complicated.

By a curious coincidence this patient also came to be treated for polypus. CASE XII.-EXTENSIVE VALVULAR DISEASE. PRACTICAL CURE WITH Arsen. iod. POLYPUS OF THE NOSE.

Wm. B-, age.26, cabinet maker, rather below middle size, but well made and well nourished, pale, came under my care May 26th, 1883, for polypus of the nose. He was treated with Thuja internally and locally, and received much benefit, the polypus diminishing much in size and ceasing to give him trouble. He continued to attend at long intervals.

May 5th, 1884.-He complained that he felt ill in himself and was low-spirited, and suffered from giddiness. He attributed it to having three stumps taken out under gas about Christmas time.

no proper sounds, all being replaced by bruits, the heart itself being much hypertrophied. I gave him Ars. iod. 3x, two grains night and morning after food, and continued the application of Thuja.

May 17th.-He expressed himself as much better generally, and gave a like report on the 31st.

On the 28th of June the improvement was still maintained, though he had not had medicine all the time. Repeat.

On July 28th he was quite free from any symptoms relating to the heart.

The first (left) sphygmographic tracing shows the aortic collapse and rebound. The other tracings, taken the same day on the right side, show this peculiarity less marked. A further sphygmogram was taken on July 26th, and the tracing was much more like a normal one. The heart sounds remained the same.

In this case the steady improvement in the heart's condition can only be attributed to the Iodide, as this was the only new element introduced into the treatment.

On the 26th of July the above tracing was taken.

CASE XIII.-DISEASE OF THE MITRAL VALVE. GREAT DEBILITY, EDEMA OF FEET. ACTION OF Iodide of arsenic.

A lady, age 58, tall, very dark, blue lips, nervous, consulted me in September, 1883. From six months old had been subject to ague. She had married rather late in life, had had no children, and had been a widow some years when she consulted me. Had never had rheumatic fever. Fifteen years before had had scarlet fever and inflammation of the lungs. Her breathing had never been quite as good since, but she only noticed distinct difficulty for six years. This had been much worse for two years. A few days before consulting me (September 17th, 1883) she had an attack of diarrhoea. This was stopped by brandy, and immediately a "cold" in the chest came on, cough hard and dry, unable to raise anything. She feels as if the windpipe were twisted and knotted, and crows with the difficulty she experiences as if she had whooping-cough. She feels very weak; is unable to walk more than a short distance, and not at all if there is a wind. The heart seems to stop and flutter. Sometimes she goes off into a kind of faint, but recovers very quickly. The feet swell about the ankles. Appetite poor; bowels confined. There is no tenderness about the larynx or trachea. The lung-sounds are feebler at left apex than right. There is a presystolic bruit.

She can sleep lying quite flat. Sleeps badly the fore part of the night, but well towards morning.

Treatment Digit. 0, one drop an hour before each meal and Arsen. iod. 1, gr. 1-20th, after food.

Three days after, she was very much better, lips less blue, expectoration easier. Much better generally. No alteration was made in the treatment. Her appetite improved, her walking powers returned, and on the 8th of October she considered herself quite well.

I will now give another case of Mitral Disease.

CASE XIV.—CONTRACTED MITRAL VALVE CLIMACTERIC SUFFERINGS. ACTION OF Arsen. iod. WITH OTHER REMEDIES.

Emma F-, age. 41, needlewoman, dark, sallow, nervous, consulted me on May 5th, 1883. She then complained of numbness and tingling in her right leg, and cramp in the right foot; numbness in arm. There was spasmodic action of the lower jaw, it closed with a jerk; (she never had had anything like this before). Had great pain in the right side of the head and burning at the vertex; the face flushed; she has pain in the back on waking. She had been ailing since the previous summer, when she had erysipelas and chronic rheumatism. The numbness had troubled her a fortnight.

The tongue was clean, bowels regular, appetite poor, sleep poor, catamenia not more than twice in the last twelve months. Pulse 102, small. She complained of her heart and breath.

On examination I found a thumping first sound, indicative of mitral stenosis, at apex. Lungs: right apex, exaggerated expiration; left apex, breathing feeble.

Treatment Arsen. iod. 3x, two grains night and morning; Ign.3, one drop three times a day.

May 19th.-Her condition has varied; has now pains all about her, pressure at the top of the head; palpitation.

Treatment Arsen. iod., night and morning; Digitalis 1, one drop three times a day.

June 20th.-Better; no pain in left arm; has sparks before the eyes. Rheumatism; pain in the back. Tongue white, bowels much confined.

The eye symptom-"Sparks before the eyes"-is a strong indication for Spigelia. I have seen similar effects occur in patients taking Spigelia in a high potency.

Treatment Spigelia 3, one drop three times a day. Arsen. iod. as before.

July 4th.- Better. Bowels regular (I have again and again noticed this effect of Spigelia in relieving constipation in cardiac patients to whom I have been giving it). She has now no sparks before the eyes, but there is much numbness in right foot and leg. Repeat.

July 21st.-Yesterday had a bad attack; has felt giddy; breathing is difficult. Has much flatulence coming upwards, bowels confined.

Treatment Lycopod. 6, vice Spigelia.

September 25th.-Very giddy at times; flatulence very troublesome; catamenia have returned. Repeat. The following month she returned, complaining of pain through the left chest, for which she received Bryonia 3, one drop in water four times a day without any other medicine. The next fortnight this pain was better, but she complained of a choking cough rising in the throat, making her sick at times; the cough came suddenly whilst talking. She had numbness down the leg, and the bowels were rather confined.

Treatment Lachesis 6, Bryonia 3; every two hours alternately.

After this she continued in much better health till January of the following year.

January 16th, 1884.-For the last fortnight she has had pain round the sacrum, coming on between 4 and 5 a.m., and preventing her sleeping after that. She trembles all over, has low spirits; pain in the side of the head. Tongue white, lips parched.

Treatment Lachesis and Bryonia.

January 30th.-Pain round the back better, but the chest is giving much trouble-this comes on when she exerts herself.

She has a creeping sensation under the skin.

I now returned to the Iodide of arsenic, giving it night and morning and continuing the Lachesis three times a day. The next report was much more favourable, and the improvement was steady and rapid till she ceased to attend on the 15th of April.

There was a steady improvement both in the heart symptoms and the general condition whilst taking the Iodide of arsenic on the first occasion, though it was never given separately, and therefore the observation is not pure. On the second occasion the improvement was much more decided, and here, as the patient was already taking Lachesis when put on Iodide of arsenic, the increased rapidity of the improvement may fairly be attributed to the latter. The case was complicated by climacteric sufferings, but the signs and symptoms of heart disease were unmistakable.

CASE XV.-MITRAL CONSTRICTION WITH ANGINOUS PAIN. Arsen. iod., Naja.

Emily T,-age 43, dark, small, housewife, was first seen on May 31st, 1882, when she gave the following report. Has pain in left side and down left arm, has had it for three or four months; it came first eight years ago, then it took the whole side.

The pain is constant and does not depend on exertion. She has palpitation, but only when she exerts herself. She always has a little cough; much expectoration in the morning, none at night; coughing makes the pain worse. She cannot lift her left arm.

Her family history is as follows. Her father died of old age; her mother of consumption when the patient was born. Three of her children and her husband have died of consumption. Patient's previous health has never been very good, but she has had no severe illnesses. A few months ago she had pain in the right side with retching, taking the strength out of her like labour pains.

The tongue was white, bowels regular,

sleep restless. The catamenia had ceased three years. She suffered from flushes; had headache at vertex and across the eyes. The pain in the arms is relieved at times by motion; the arm swells at times. Examination of the heart showed the existence of stenosis of the mitral valve. Bryonia and subsequently Spigelia failed to give substantial relief.

June 28th.-Arm not any better.

I now gave her the Arsen. iod. 3x, 2 grains three times a day, and this, as generally happened, soon told beneficially on the general health, causing some improvement in the pain.

July 12th.-Feeling better generally, pain not quite so bad, breath much the same. Repeat.

Feeling better she did not return for six weeks.

August 23rd.-Arm has been better, but it is very painful again to-day. Repeat.

September 13th.-Arm better at times; for a few days it has been bad, it feels cold, aching is continuous.

Treatment Naja 6, every three hours. Arsen. iod. 3x, night and morning.

The next report was that the arm was much better. Repeat.

This was her last attendance. In this case the improvement was initiated by Arsen.iod. alone, but it did not give complete relief; this was left for Naja to accomplish.

It is remarkable how frequently disease of the heart is met with in patients with a strong consumptive history. This was exemplified in the case of Emily T-, and also in the one I will now relate. The power of Arsen.iod. to relieve many cases of phthisis may account for its wide range of action in cases of heart disease.

CASE XVI.-MITRAL INCOMPETENCE, DILATATION OF LEFT AURICLE, AND HYPERTROPHY OF RIGHT SIDE OF HEART.

Salome B, age. 38, single, housekeeper, dark, blue lips, attended at the L. H. Hospital on August 30th, 1882.

She complained that she felt ill in the morning, and could hardly raise herself from her pillow. Two years before she had "congestion of the liver" and now she feels just as she did then; she has a heavy pain in the left side, depression of spirits. She gets no rest, comes over faint, especially on walking. Has headache across the forehead and vertex on waking. Tongue clean, appetite poor, bowels regular, sleep bad, catamenia scanty, regular.

She has never been strong; her mother died of consumption; also one brother and one sister. Her father is living, but in poor health.

Examination.-Has scar of ulcerated gland on right side of root of neck. Lungs: apices clear. Heart: apex beat not visible, it is felt in the fifth space three inches to left of sternum. Vertical dullness begins in the middle of the second space. Transverse dullness at the level of the fourth costal cartilage extends one inch to the right and three inches to the left of the sternum. In the mitral area is a soft systolic bruit, heard also sometimes in the third space. The second sound is accentuated and occasionally reduplicated in the pulmonary area.

Treatment Arsen. iod. 3x, night and morning; Digitalis 1, three times a day.

The following fortnight (September 13th) she attended again.

September 13th.-The pain is rather better and also the palpitation; but she has taken a cold and (as is usually the case with her when she takes cold) had lost her voice. Repeat.

October 4th.-Better generally, voice better. She complains, however, that the medicine (Digitalis) makes her ill; it seems to make her heart palpitate. The palpitation and pain are worse than last time; she has pain between the shoulders. She has had some annoyance during the week.

R Ignat. 1x, four times a day. Arsen. iod. as before.

October 25th.-Not nearly so much pain; less palpitation. She has a sinking sensation sometimes.

This was her last attendance. There was a great improvement in her general condition as well as in the special symptoms. I ascribe the chief share of this to the Iodide. I am inclined to believe the patient was correct in attributing the aggravation of her symptoms to the Digitalis, and certainly the substitution of Ignatia was followed by very marked improvement.

Rheumatism and Chorea are fruitful causes of heart disease. In the case next to be related there was a history of epilepsy and stammering (which is itself a choreic condition) previous to the heart attack.

CASE XVII.-MITRAL CONSTRICTION IN PATIENT PREVIOUSLY EPILEPTIC.

Chas. H. S.-age. 14, errand boy, dark eyes, light hair. This patient was treated by me in 1882 for epilepsy. The only medicine he received was Stramonium 3. I did not see him again until January, 1884. I then learned that he had never had a fit since his previous attendance. He stammered badly. This had been the case since he was three years old. It came on during dentition.

January 25th, 1884.-He now complains of pain at the heart and of being weak and nervous. If he breathes hard it catches him and he has to fight for breath. The pain is sharp, pinching, and constant. He is short of breath ongoing upstairs. All this came on nine months before, the pain preceding the breathlessness. It came quite suddenly; he was running to his work and the pain stopped him. Tongue white; bowels regular; sleep sound. He always has headache over the left eye.

I found on listening over the apex beat the characteristic thump of obstructed mitral; there was a faint venous hum in the neck. The heart's action was not regular. The pulse was very small.

Treatment Arsen. iod. night and morning, and Digit. 1, one pilule three times a day.

He came back in a fortnight feeling much better. Has only had two attacks of the heart-pain in the fortnight. His stammering was rather worse. He received another supply of medicine.

I will now relate a case of heart affection of a gouty nature.

CASE XVIII.—IRRITABLE WEAK HEART IN A GOUTY SUBJECT. HISTORY OF OVER-STRAIN; ACTION OF Arsen. iod.

The patient was a lady, age. 66, short, very stout, florid. As a child she was delicate; in middle life her health was good except that she suffered almost constantly from supraorbital neuralgia. She had lived in India some years, and had very good health except very slight attacks of fever, which seemed to relieve her of the neuralgic pains. In

1854 she had cholera in Edinburgh. Had been a great walker.

In 1884, when she consulted me, I made the following notes:- Has gouty concretions about the joints of her hands, and her feet are deformed in the same way. Her present illness dates from six years back; she was climbing a hill in Scotland, and she felt at the time she had done too much; she thought she never would have got her breath again; she has never been right in her breathing since.

After this she had a cold and cough for six weeks; it is unusual for her to take cold-she loves air and open windows. (When I saw her she had had a cold in the head; this had left the head and gone to the chest). She complains of great dyspnoea in the night, and whistling in the chest, which keeps her awake; has a sensation about the heart as if something were nipping her there-this is confined to an area about the size of a crown-piece; then she feels as if passing away, but recovers if she is quite still. At times she has a sensation of fullness, as if something in the chest would burst. Exertion or worry will bring on cough. There is no swelling of the feet. Poor appetite. I found slight wheezing here and there in the lungs.

On examining the chest I found the second sound of the heart accentuated at all areas, the first sound very faint except at the apex; there was no bruit.

I gave her Carbo v. 6, every three hours for three days, and there was considerable improvement, which, however, was not maintained. I then gave her Kali carb. 6, an hour before meals, and Arsen. iod.1, gr. 1/10, in water, immediately after food. The improvement was marked and rapid; she could move about with more comfort, and the appetite improved. Four days after this I gave her the Iodide 3x, 1 gr. three times a day after food, by itself.

She kept much better and was able to leave town soon after.

Quite recently (1894) I learned from a

daughter of this patient that she died a few years ago of cancer in the left breast.

Needless to say, there are numbers of cases which are not perceptibly influenced by the Iodide. Homoeopathy has specifics for patients not for diseases, hence a strict attention to symptomatology is the only safe rule in this as in all departments of our art, as the case next to be related will exemplify.

CASE XIX.-IMMENSELY ENLARGED, DISPLACED HEART; VALVULAR DISEASE; INDIGESTION. GREAT RELIEF FROM VARIOUS REMEDIES.

It is notable how frequently cardiac patients complain more than anything else of indigestion. It was the principal thing the patient, James T., complained of before the attack which brought him under my care. It was the chief trouble in two of the cases still to be mentioned. In the case I am now going to relate, that of Mrs. W., an octogenarian, the strictest attention to dietetic rules was absolutely necessary in order to keep her in comfort.

This patient had survived a number of illnesses, including a right-side pleurisy many years before, which had left her with a shrunken lung and curved spine and a displacement of the heart to the right. The heart was greatly hypertrophied, and there were murmurs to be heard at every orifice, a double aortic, loud systolic at mitral and tricuspid. The heart's action was very irregular, the arteries hard and tortuous.

I attended her through a variety of illnesses, diphtheritic sore throat, bronchitis on various occasions, influenza with bronchitis, minor urinary troubles and psoriasis. The condition of the heart dominated everything. There was great swelling of the feet, which varied in degree at different times. But her chief trouble was indigestion and flatulence; the smallest transgression was pretty sure to be visited by an "attack" in the early hours of the morning. The "attack" was a feeling of faintness, a sensation that she was "going," violent pain at times in the region of the heart's apex, great oppression, the symptoms being relieved after a greater or less time by a copious flow of colorless urine. Every time I was called to her in one of these attacks she thought she was dying, and was almost angry with me because I refused to confirm her prognosis and pronounce the viaticum.

Aurum metallicum in the 30th or 1m gave prompt relief to this feeling of impending death and kept her reconciled to life for long periods at a time.

Kali carb. in the same potencies gave her great help when the attacks came on between 2 and 5 A.M., and when there was a cough with aggravation at those hours. After an attack, when there was much palpitation and breathlessness with heart discomfort, Baryt. carb.5 and 30, gave much relief. On occasional courses of these medicines she was kept in tolerable health for long periods. When I first began to treat her I gave the Iodide of arsenic with some benefit; but it was not nearly so marked as that from the more definitely indicated remedies in higher powers. Aurum 1m (Boericke & Tafel, or F. C.), had the most prompt action when the sensation of impending death was marked.

I will place beside this case another of extensively damaged heart in an aged patient, in which there were practically no symptoms referable to the heart itself, and consequently no call for special treatment.

CASE XX.-EXTENSIVELY DAMAGED HEART AND ARTERIES FULLY COMPENSATED AND GIVING RISE TO NO SYMPTOMS.

A stalwart octogenarian, Andrew M., came to my out-patient clinic at the Homoeopathic Hospital in the summer of 1882, complaining of rheumatic pains in various parts.

Two years before he had been laid up for five weeks with rheumatic fever, and for a short time after that he had been troubled with shortness of breath on going up stairs, but had got over that, and had not been troubled with any heart symptoms since. His irregular pulse, sharp and hard, and hard tortuous arteries at once told me that damage had been done. Here are two of his sphygmograms, pressure 4 ounces.

Examination of the heart showed the following:

There was visible pulsation in the carotids, the apex beat was in the fifth interspace, 3 1/2 inches to the left of the sternum, and the transverse dullness extended from 1/4 inch on the right of the sternum 4 inches to the left.

Vertical dullness began at the lower border of the third rib. No bruits were audible, but there was at the apex the peculiar thumping first sound which indicates mitral stenosis, this being followed by a sharp second. Over the aortic and pulmonary areas the first sound was inaudible, the second being sharply accentuated, the accentuation being most marked in the aortic area. An exaggerated second means increased backward pressure on the heart, and in the case of the aortic valve, it is generally the prelude to aortic incompetence and regurgitation. When the aorta has been affected, either by acute inflammation, as in fevers, or by chronic degeneration, it loses a certain amount of elasticity, and becomes permanently dilated under the force of the heart's beats. When this has taken place the rebound of the column of blood after the systole is more sudden, and produces the accentuation of the second sound in the aortic area, such as was present in this case. The defect was compensated by hypertrophy.

The rheumatic symptoms gradually subsided under Bryonia and Colchicum, and finally, Pulsatilla 3, which last did more for him than any other remedy. It removed, after the other medicines had failed, swelling, pain and numbness of the hands across the metacarpal joints, worse in the morning on rising, and left him practically well. The only symptoms he had during the course of the treatment referable to the heart were temporary giddiness and buzzing in the ears.

In this case I did not think it necessary to alarm the patient by explaining to him the condition of his heart, as I believed it would last him as long as the rest of his body.

I will now give the particulars of a case which first came under my care as one of "indigestion."

CASE XXI.-MITRAL DISEASE WITH ATTACKS OF SYNCOPE. ACTION OF Ignatia.

Mr. J. W., a tradesman, who had done work about my house, consulted me occasionally for an "indigestion" he was troubled with from time to time. The first time was in February, 1888, he being then 38 years old. The symptoms of his indigestion were weight at the epigastrium after food, tenderness to pressure, and drowsiness after meals. These symptoms were quickly removed by Bryonia. He also suffered frequently from headache, tightness at the chest, pain between the shoulders, and at times a cough. His pulse was somewhat frequent, but there was nothing sufficiently remarkable about it to make me suspect anything wrong with his heart.

On April 13th, 1889, I was summoned to see him in the greatest urgency. After a good deal of worry he had been suddenly seized with violent palpitation and faintness, and when I saw him he was in a death-like faint, pallid, with purple lips, and icy cold; in fact he was in a very grave condition of cardiac syncope; the pulse was weak and slow. On examining his chest, I found the heart enlarged, and a mitral systolic bruit present. I put on his tongue a dose of Ignatia 1m (Boericke and Tafel) and repeated it frequently, and he soon revived sufficiently to enable me to take him home in a cab (for he was at his place of business at the time of the seizure). On examining him more at leisure, I found the systolic bruit (which was soft) was audible over the apex, and also over the left auricle. The condition was one of mitral incompetence with hypertrophy.

I now learned that for some time past he had noticed a shortness of breath on going up stairs, and three months before he had turned faint suddenly, and was compelled to sit down. I continued the Ignatia, and I may say that ever since that time it has been a very good friend to my patient. He never goes anywhere without a bottle of pilules of the medicine in the same strength, and whenever he has any sensation of weakness about the heart, whether induced by worry, or by over-exertion, a few doses soon put him right. He has never had a fully developed attack again. He is fair, and of a very sensitive temperament, and easily affected by worry, but active and muscularly strong.

To return now to my journal:-

April 14th.-Had a slight attack in the evening after talking. Dreamed much in the night; short breath on going up stairs; head feels rather light; feet rather colder. Continue Ignatia.

April 16th.-Headache in occiput; fluttering sensation in left chest; faint trembling after waking; a little fever; much flatus downwards; thirst; lips dry. Arsenicum 1m every two hours. Ignatia if required.

April 17th.- Went for a walk yesterday, but could not go far. Dreamed much all night- muddled dreams. Tongue white; still thirsty; bowels rather confined; occipital headache on waking; tremor at heart. Repeat.

I need not follow out the case from day to day. There was another slight attack on the 20th, but by the end of the month the patient was able to return to his work. He had occasionally drawing or digging pain in his left side, and at times a sharp pain, and headache remained troublesome. At one time he described it as a "floating weight" at the vertex. This was relieved by Act. rac. 1. On May 8th he complained of feeling a weight at epigastrium after food, sinking sensation coming on after dinner, and constipation. He received Sulph. 30, one pilule three times a day. After this he was practically well, Sulphur and Ignatia being the chief remedies he required.

Early in the following year he had influenza very badly, with pneumonia and pleurisy of the left side. The heart was not directly involved. The bruit was heard, though faintly. Sulphur was his chief remedy on this occasion. At present he is in very good health. If he over-exerts himself, especially when at work on great heights, as the roofs of London houses, he is reminded that he has a heart. I examined his chest quite recently, and found this condition :-

Apex beat not felt. Area of cardiac dullness extends 2 1/2 inches to left of sternal edge. In pulmonary and aortic areas the first sound is soft; at the mitral area no bruit is heard, but the first sound is impure. This shows that the mitral valve has been restored to competence, though not to its normal state. The sharp, clear sound of the closing of healthy valves is wanting.

This patient has never had rheumatic fever, or any illness to which the state of his heart could be traced. He has always been temperate. Eleven years ago he was very nearly killed by a brick falling on his head from a building in course of erection; but this is the only illness of consequence that he remembers.

The above sphygmogram was taken on March 21, 1893, pressure 3 1/2 ounces.

The foregoing cases, chosen out of a large number, will, I think, suffice to prove that valvular disease of the heart is often curable under Homoeopathic treatment; and when the valves are beyond repair and the balance of the organ lost, much may still be done by Homoeopathy to give power to the heart and restore its equilibrium.

Chapter 4 THE ACTION OF THYROIDIN IN DISEASES OF THE HEART.[The Action of Thyroidin] THE allopathic school of medicine has very much to learn in the matter of dosage. It invariably begins at the wrong end of the scale. The recent introduction of preparations of the Thyroid Gland of the sheep furnishes a case in point. These various preparations (which have received the generic name of Thyroidin, being in nature practically identical) were given at first in such massive doses that a large number of pathogenetic effects were produced, and, among others, in several cases, fatal fainting. A collection of these effects has been made by me, and will be found recorded in Volume XXIX. (1894) of the Homoeopathic World.

From the June number (p.254) I will transcribe the symptoms relating to the heart and circulation produced in cases of allopathic over-dosing, and also some cured symptoms. The latter are marked with the small circle "o" placed at the beginning of the symptom refer to the authorities given in the May number (pp. 202-216).

HEART AND CIRCULATION.-On trying to

walk uphill died suddenly from cardiac failure.1

While stooping to put on her shoes she "fainted" and died in half an hour.1

Two fainting attacks.2

One patient showed extraordinary symptoms after the injection. The skin became so livid as to be almost blue-black.3

(Degeneration of heart muscle in animals.)4

Increased pulse-rate.5

A systolic cardiac murmur was less loud after the treatment than before.7

Complained occasionally of a feeling of faintness, not occurring particularly after the injections.8

Sensations of faintness and nausea.8

Frequent fainting fits.8

Palpitation on stooping.9

Pulse 64, regular, compressible.9

On one occasion, after exerting herself more than she had done for a long time previously, she "suddenly became extremely breathless and livid, and felt as if she were dying. Rest in recumbent position and the prompt administration of stimulants restored her, but she seems very narrowly to have escaped the fate of two of Dr. Murray's patients."10

Pulse rose to 112. 16

Tachycardia. 17,23

Fatal syncope.18

Weakness of heart's action.29

Tachycardia and ready excitability of the heart persisting for several days after the feeding was stopped. 18

Relaxation of arterioles. 18

In lupus of face heat and red, angry appearance removed. 27

Death, with all the symptoms of angina pectoris. 18

Rapid pulsation, with inability to lie down in bed. 21

Jumping sensation at heart. 21

FEVER.-Flushing, with nausea.

Flushing, with loss of consciousness. 1

Skin became so livid as to be almost blue-black. 3

Face flushed. 5

Rise of temperature, 100 degree F. 5

Profuse perspiration on least exertion. 6

Always felt hot, and had a sensation of sickness after the injections. 7

Felt better and warmer. 11

Flushing of upper part of body and pains in back. 11

Temperature never rose above 99 degree she felt feverish and thirsty. 13

Temperature rose to 100 degree but F., and remained there several days; pulse 112. 16

Rise of temperature; diaphoresis. 17, 18, 23

From this it will be seen how powerful is the action of this drug (which I think may be fitly called a Sarcode) on the heart and circulation. If allopaths would only consent to learn the homoeopathic method of attenuating medicines, they might avoid all the risks of fatal over-dosing which they (or rather their patients) have to run whenever a new drug is introduced. However, to Homoeopathy belongs the blessed function of turning to good account for mankind some of the havoc done by allopathy. To the homoeopath all these violent heart symptoms mark the medicine out as a great heart remedy, and I will now give a few cases in which I have been able to turn this indication to good account.

The first patient for whom I prescribed it was a young woman with a highly neurotic history presenting all the symptoms of incipient "Graves' Disease" or Exophthalmic Goitre.

There was prominence of the eyes, enlargement of the thyroid gland, and rapid action of the heart (tachycardia) together with much heart pain and inability to lie flat in bed. This was one of those distressing neurotic cases in which there is a very great amount of suffering without any serious organic change. The suffering is perfectly real, but the patient is abnormally sensitive, and often imaginative, and generally gains little sympathy from her medical attendants.

The action of Thyroidin was most satisfactory in this case, and the potency used-the 3rd decimal, i.e. 1/1000th of a grain of the thyroid extract to each grain of the preparation-showed how needless is all the allopathic over-dosing.

I will now give the history of the case, as written out for me by the then House Physician, Dr. Lambert.
CASE XXII.-HEART PAIN, WITH RAPID ACTION, AND SYMPTOMS OF EXOPHTHALMIC GOITRE IN NEUROTIC SUBJECT. CURE WITH Thyroidin.

Eleanor N., age, 17, was admitted to the London Homoeopathic Hospital, under Dr. Clarke, on October 10th, 1893. She had always been very nervous and had had chorea, and suffered much from palpitation.

Since Christmas, 1892, she had had attacks of hystero-epilepsy, which, in the first place, followed a chill. The fits were as frequent as seven in a day at first, and recurred daily. The frequency of the attacks diminished till, latterly, they had occurred only before the menstrual period. The fits used to last half-an-hour, and were preceded by swelling of the limbs and face, which sometimes occured without the subsequent fit. She used to bite her tongue in the fits.

Besides these attacks she complained of pains in the legs, back, and head-the headache being occipital, and in the vertex; also that her throat swelled at times, so that she had to loosen her clothes. The catamenia had been absent for four months, till the last time, which was excessive. She always had a good deal of pain at that time, especially in the left ovarian region, which was always tender to pressure.

Her family history was good with the exception that one brother was epileptic.

On admission, she was in a low, despondent state of mind, evidently very neurotic. Her eyes were staring and prominent. The heart sounds were weak, but no bruit present. Pulse was 120. Her legs were so weak that she could not stand.

There was no very great enlargement

of the thyroid gland, but there was distinct fullness of the neck.

and caused palpitation. She slept badly, and used, previously to admission, to take hypnotics regularly. The bowels were always constipated, and the stools hard and painful. Sulph. 30 was given every four hours, and on the 14th Lachesis 12 was substituted, under which she improved somewhat, and slept decidedly better. On October 18th Sac.-Lact. was given and continued till the 25th. Crocus 30 was then ordered on the indication—"a sensation of jumping at the heart." It was continued till November 1st, but it did not remove the symptom.

Up to this point there had certainly been improvement in the patient's condition, but it was very slow. She still had frequent headache and a rapid pulse, and her legs were very weak, though with assistance she was got up daily. She was sleeping well, but needed several pillows, as she could not lie down flat. The bowels were never moved without enemata. She was now put on Thyroidin 3x, gr. ij, three times a day, and from that time forward improvement was marked. On November 4th she could lie down flat. November 15th she could walk much better, but not alone. November 29th the headache had quite ceased, and she was better in every way. December 6th she could walk alone quite well, and the bowels acted normally for the first time, and continued to do at first every second day, and then every day without any trouble.

Her mental condition was also markedly improved, and the prominence of the eyeballs disappeared. She was kept in hospital a month longer to prevent relapse, and before Christmas was perfectly well.

I will next relate a case from private practice in which the exophthalmic symptoms were more fully developed. Thyroidin in a higher potency acted very promptly, even relieving acute inflammatory symptoms induced by an intercurrent attack of influenza.
CASE XXIII.-HYPERTROPHY WITH

TACHYCARDIA, AND ATTACKS OF ANGINA PECTORIS. ACTION OF Thyroidin.

Miss C., 35, has been under my care occasionally for a number of years. She has an exceedingly bad family history, nearly all the members of her mother's family having died suddenly of heart disease. At the age of 13 the patient had scarlatina, followed by inflammation of one of her ears; some bone came away from the mastoid process. She became deaf till she took influenza, during which she had another attack of inflammation which had the effect of perfectly restoring her hearing on that side. At the age of 17 she suffered from enlarged tonsils, and had them removed.

Afterwards she suffered from enlarged thyroid gland, and attacks of palpitation. In 1891 she had influenza, which left her liable to palpitation on the least exertion. In September of this year she had a pulse of 120, attacks of pain in the left side, with sensation as if the heart would burst out of the chest. Lying on the left side was impossible. There was no bruit or evidence of any affection of the heart's valves. Under Spongia 30 she got better of this attack.

In December, 1893, a mental shock-the sudden death of her mother from heart disease-again brought on an attack of pain and palpitation, this was followed by another acute attack of influenza, with pains all over the body, especially the feet and ankles. At times the attacks of palpitation would come on in the middle of the night, compelling her to jump out of bed.

Examination of the heart showed that it was greatly enlarged. The area of dullness was much increased; the apex beat was far to the left of its normal position. There was tenderness over the apex beat, and this was the seat of the pain. No evidence of any valve involvement. Thyroid gland distinctly enlarged; eyes not particularly prominent. When the rheumatic symptoms of the influenza had subsided, inflammation of the ear supervened. The patient suffered excessive pain which the usual remedies did not relieve very much; the pain coming in paroxysms, and lasting some hours, being worse from 1 to 5 a.m.

The ear had begun to discharge freely.

Taking into account her general state, the thyroid enlargement, heart pain, palpitation, and flushes of heat from which the patient suffered, I prescribed on February 17th Thyroidin 30, a few globules dissolved in water; a teaspoonful every two hours.

After five doses she lost the pain completely, and for the first time slept a night through. The following night she had some pain, but it did not commence till 7 a.m. Pulse much quieter.

February 21st.-Very bad earache last night.

Treatment Puls. 30 every two hours.

February 22nd.-No pain in night, had some during the day. Repeat.

February 23nd.-Earache all night; some discharge; worse in warm room.

I now returned to Thyroidin, which I gave every hour.

February 25th.-Ear better; had three hours pain on night of 23rd, but none since.

On the 27th the heart was very troublesome again. The monthly period was due but had not come on; she had a sensation as if the heart stopped. I gave Pulsatilla again, and afterwards, Psorinum, but without much relief; and on March 3rd I returned to Thyroidin, which relieved the heart at once.

The period came on the same day. Since then the heart has given the patient very little trouble, and when she has felt it a few doses of Thyroidin have sufficed to put it right again.

Here is an acute case to which I have

already alluded in Chapter II.
CASE XXIV.- ACUTE VALVULAR AFFECTION OF THE HEART WITH SEVERE
HEART PAIN. CURATIVE ACTION OF Thyroidin.

Sydney C., 24 porter, fair, sanguine temperament, robust- looking, was admitted to the hospital November 15th, 1893. Three or four years before he had had pleurisy. He is subject to attacks of pleurisy whenever he takes cold. Three months ago he was taken ill with pains all over, chiefly in his joints; since then he had been unable to work. On admission he complained of pains in the region of the heart, as if the heart were being squeezed; severe headaches, shooting pains in forehead and vertex chiefly, sometimes also in occiput. Burning pain round left costal margin, worse after drinking; also about half an hour after eating, pain in epigastrium to the left side, as if the food stuck there. Shooting pain across cardiac region and under left shoulder. On stooping and lifting, pain across lumbar region.

Appetite good; has much flatulence upward; water brash, very sour, comes on soon after drinking. Bowels regular as a rule.

Has palpitation, chiefly at night, caused by any slight noise. Orthopnoea: if he lies down the squeezing sensation at the heart comes on. Dyspnoea on exertion.

State of the heart.-Apex beat visible in fifth space in nipple line. Impulse weak. Systolic bruit heard in aortic area, and all along the sternum and in tricuspid region. Second sound weak. Mitral soft, blowing, systolic murmur very faint.

Eruption of acne on left side of chest. Pupils both very much dilated. Urine alkaline, no albumen, copious phosphates.

Treatment Cactus 30 every four hours.

Later examinations of the heart gave the following results:- November 22nd.- Systolic bruit not so loud in aortic area as in left auricular area.

November 27th.-No aortic bruit heard to-day, no mitral bruit, both sounds indistinct and muffled.

November 30th.-Faint systolic heard in pulmonary region; first sound very impure in mitral area, inaudible in aortic.

December 14th.-First sound very muffled; inaudible in aortic and pulmonary areas.

This was the last examination made. The attack was of a rheumatic nature, involving the heart, and complicated with flatulent indigestion.

Apparently from another patient in the ward, with fever, cough, backache and headache, his other pains being intensified at the same time.

December 4th.-Flatulence very bad during the night, causing much pain in the chest.

Treatment Carbo.-veg. 12, every two hours during the night.

After this he slept better, and was free from indigestion for some days; but still there was at times a good deal of flatulence and acid risings; and palpitation waking him in the night.

On December 27th, guided largely by persistent rapidity of the pulse, and faintness of which he frequently complained on waking, I put him on Thyroidin 3x, gr. ij, three times a day.

The heart pains quickly subsided, but the flatulence continued, and I gave Carbo.-veg. when required, in addition to the Thyroidin.

December 30th.-Pulse diminished much in frequency. Is better, except for flatulence.

Treatment Carbo.-an. 12. Stop Thyroidin.

January 3rd, 1894.-Flatulence better. Pain under heart again, and round left side.

Repeat Thyroidin.

January 5th.-Better than he has been for a long time. Less flatulence. Still sour water brash.

January 6th.-No pains at all. Flatulence better.

January 10th.-Flatulence troublesome again. Pulse 84.

Treatment Carbo.-an. 12.

January 13th.-Flatulence better.

He was discharged practically well on January 15th. The Thyroidin had more marked effect on the cardiac distress than any other medicine given, and I have no doubt greatly expedited the patient's recovery. He was quite well enough to return to work when he left the hospital.

Chapter 5 PALPITATION AND FAINTING.

[Palpitation and Fainting] Of all the symptoms connected with the heart the most common is undoubtedly palpitation. It is a frequent accompaniment of actual disease of the heart, but it is safe to say that in nine cases out of ten in which it occurs there is no discoverable structural alteration of the organ itself.

The frequent, forcible and often painful pulsation of the heart coming in paroxysms depends on a disturbance in the nervous control of the heart. It is occasioned, as is very well known, by a variety of emotions, by over-exertion, by evil habits, by over indulgence in tobacco and coffee, by injudicious drugging, by faulty dress.

In this chapter I shall not consider those cases in which palpitation occurs as a result of organic disease, nor those (dealt with in the preceding chapter) in which it forms one of the phenomena of exophthalmic goitre, or the condition called "Tachycardia" (rapid heart), where it is a permanent feature. I shall include here only those cases in which there is a liability to attacks on slight provocation, and those in which attacks seem to come on without any provocation whatever.

Women are much more liable to be affected with this form of heart disturbance than men, and the times when it is most troublesome are puberty and the climacteric. No doubt the difference in the organisation and temperament of the two sexes has much to do with this, but there is another factor which is accountable for a vast deal of the heart-suffering of women, and that is-dress. As soon as girls begin to grow up they are compelled to wear corsets, which, if they do not actually constrict the lower segment of the chest, do prevent the proper movement of the chest wall and hinder proper development. Nature has made the lowest ribs free to expand and dilate with the exigencies of breathing; dressmakers have infringed on this by substituting a rigid wall. The lungs not having sufficient room for their natural motion press on the heart and incommode its action. Not having proper room in which to dilate, it makes up for inefficient action by over-rapid action, and thus there is an attack of palpitation whenever any unusual demand is made on the heart and lungs. I need hardly add that when a good meal is added to the contents of the corset, the crowded state of matters is much increased.

The figure of a woman demands a somewhat different style of dress from that of a man, but the part on which the pressure ought to be put is the hips-the part which shelves outwards from the crest of the hip-bone to the prominence of the thigh bone (great trochanter) over the hip-joint.

No amount of pressure can do harm there. But the free ribs must be left free, and corsets should be made of some material which is not rigid but elastic, and which will allow the natural motions of the chest wall to take place. The "Curetta" corset and those made by the Jaeger company fulfil these conditions.

In the same connection may be mentioned another cause of palpitation, and this is, indigestion. Many people think they have heart disease when they have nothing more than indigestion. The heart and stomach are under the control of the same nerve, so that any injury to one is often felt sympathetically by the other. The stomach lies within the arch of the free ribs; anything therefore which lessens this space interferes with the stomach and cramps it for room, and is sufficient to cause indigestion. The heart and the stomach are only separated by the diaphragm, hence any over-distention of the stomach, whether by flatulence or food, is very apt to give rise to heart symptoms.

In young men one of the most frequent causes of palpitation is indulgence in tobacco. Tobacco has four favourite seats on which it expends the brunt of its action-the nervous system, the heart, the eye and the throat. It may be one of these only, or it may be a combination. I have seen the most abject terror of death in connection with disturbed heart's action, produced by excessive smoking.

Another very fruitful cause of it (and this applies to both sexes) is the practice of vicious habits which are generally learned at school. In these cases it is one of many other symptoms, but often the leading one. It does not often lead to organic change, but it does sometimes. In one case, in a young man where there was both valvular defect and hypertrophy, under a prolonged course of Natrum mur. the valvular defect disappeared and also the palpitation with other subjective symptoms.

When the cause is known and removable, the clear indication is to remove it. But in these cases much help may be given by homoeopathy to relieve the sufferings entailed in breaking off old habits and stimulants. For instance, Nux vomica and Arsenicum will often enable tobacco devotees to break off their habit; Nux, Sulphur, Lachesis, China, and again

Arsenicum with several other medicines will weaken or destroy the craving for alcohol in drunkards.

But there are many cases in which the cause is not to be removed. In naturally sensitive persons, when the least excitement of any kind will set up palpitation, Ignatia and the serpent poisons are invaluable. Climacteric palpitations (which though far more common in women than in men are not by any means confined to one sex), are very frequently removed by medicines.

CASE XXV.-CLIMACTERIC PALPITATION CURED BY Glonoin. Glonoin, the medicine prepared from Nitroglycerine, is one of the glories of homoeopathy. Almost as soon as the substance was discovered Constantine Hering, of Philadelphia, procured some and proved it. Soon afterwards Dudgeon and others in this country further tested its powers by taking it themselves. In these experiments the power of the drug on the heart and circulation was fully manifested, and it was not long before it was turned to very good account in practice. The allopaths have recently adopted the discovery, and even adopted the first Hahnemannian dilution of the medicine. The history of the discovery they are careful not to mention, and naturally enough they have not adopted the name Hering coined out of its chemical formula-they adhere to its longer title, Nitro-glycerine.

But to come to my case. The patient, a lady, just at the commencement of the menopause, was suddenly seized one day with violent palpitation, together with throbbing in the blood-vessels all over the body, and more especially the head. She was for the time so ill that she was unable to do anything, and had some trouble in getting to her bed-room.

A few doses of Glonoin quieted the storm in a very short time, and it never afterwards recurred in the same violence. When it did recur Glonoin soon relieved the patient.

Belladonna is another valuable medicine in cases of excited heart action. Probably Belladonna would have helped this patient if Glonoin had not been discovered, but not so promptly. The following case shows its power very well.

CASE XXVI.-PALPITATION IN AN ATTACK OF ACUTE ILLNESS. Belladonna.

A lady, 56, in the course of an attack of broncho-pneumonia was seized with a fit of palpitation of great severity; she could not lie down in bed, her face was flushed intensely, and she was in the greatest distress. The heart was evidently beyond the control of its usual nervous controlling influences.

Belladonna 30 was given at once. Almost immediately the attack moderated. A few more doses at frequent intervals put an end to it entirely.

CASE XXVII.-PALPITATION FROM WORRY. Ignatia.

Another patient about the climacteric suffered from distressing attacks of palpitation when anything occurred to give her annoyance or worry.

When things went smoothly nothing of the kind occurred. But when once set up the heart irritability continued a long time. I gave her Ignatia 30. This rapidly relieved the condition, and made her less susceptible to the effects of worry afterwards.

FAINTING.

Syncope or fainting is another common accompaniment of heart affections, but it is much more frequently met within patients who have no organic affection of the heart at all. The amount of danger attending it depends on whether or not organic disease is present, and on the cause which has given rise to the attack. Fainting from violent emotional disturbance may prove fatal even without the presence of organic disease; but in the vast majority of cases fainting is a temporary affection rapidly recovered from. I have known fainting caused in workpeople whose employment necessitated the use of charcoal fires. After a time they would become habituated to breathing the fumes; but at first it brought on fainting attacks.

A faint means that for some reason or other the heart's action has become too feeble to send a sufficient amount of blood to the brain; and this results in temporary loss of consciousness and muscular power.

The cause of the collapse may be of nervous origin, as some sudden shock or emotion; or fainting may arise from some defect or weakness of the heart itself.

Many cases of fainting are in reality slight attacks of epilepsy; and catalepsy is responsible for many others. In the latter attacks there is some element of the trance condition. The patient becomes cold and rigid, and though unable to move is not entirely unconscious. In these cases and in many others Moschus will be found a remedy of the greatest value. And the value of Moschus is not by any means confined to the cases in which no organic affection is found : it will relieve fainting, and the tendency to it in many cases of badly damaged heart.

Chapter 7 ANGINA PECTORIS.[Angina Pectoris]

LIKE every other organ and part of the body which contains nerves, the heart may be the seat of neuralgic pain. Heart pains may vary in intensity from something so slight that it hardly merits the name of pain to the intensest agony of the worst forms of Angina Pectoris or "Breast Pang." This latter may occur in connection with actual organic disease of the heart and its vessels (instances of which have been already given), or it may be a pure neuralgia. In either form it may prove fatal in a paroxysm. A good many years ago I was called to make a post mortem examination of a man about 50 who had been found dead in the street in a doubled-up condition. I found the heart rigidly contracted and nothing else about him to account for death. The man had died of heart spasm. This was a case of pure Angina Pectoris, the muscle and vessels of the heart being healthy.

Compare with this the case of a gentleman who fell down whilst walking home across one of the parks. He was able to get up again and finish his walk, but had very much pain at the heart, and breathlessness, until he died ten days later. In this case there was extensive fatty degeneration of the heart wall and degeneration of the coronary arteries of the heart, which were almost occluded with the products of disease.

The disease which was revealed at the post mortem was quite sufficient to account for the heart failure; but it was of such a nature that no examination of the heart before death could have declared its presence, though the symptoms pointed to it. In case of this kind, as in many others, the symptoms are not only the safest but the only guide to diagnosis.

CASE XXXI.-ANGINA PECTORIS OF VACCINAL ORGAN. CURED BY Thuja.
Neuralgias of the heart do not arise (any more than other neuralgias) from

nothing, even when there is no discoverable organic disease present. Nerve pains are symptoms of some defect of nutrition or the presence of some subtle poison, e.g., malarial or other fever poisons, or one or other of the chronic miasms of Hahnemann, or the poison of vaccinia.

The case I am now about to relate was one of the last class. The patient, a lady about middle life, had been vaccinated about a dozen times. She suffered from terrible attacks of neuralgia of head and face, more or less periodic, and at times from intense attacks of angina pectoris, generally coming on in the night, waking her out of sleep.

She received benefit from a number of remedies, but it was not until I realized the vaccinal origin of the malady and gave the patient Thuja in an exceedingly high potency that the attacks were got rid of altogether. A single dose of Thuja, after producing a severe aggravation, put an end to the attacks.

It required more than a single dose, however, to get rid of the vaccinal diathesis; for the same patient developed tumours in first one and then the other breast which caused her great alarm as she feared at first that they were cancerous. I strongly deprecated the idea of operation, and fortunately in this I was seconded by an allopathic doctor who saw the patient (she lived at the time in the country away from any homoeopath). Under medicines, and Thuja among the chief, the tumours disappeared and the patient regained a measure of health and strength to which she had been for many years a stranger.

Influenza has been responsible for many deaths from sudden heart failure with angina pectoris. I have seen a number of cases of angina caused by influenza, but happily they all recovered.

CASE XXXII.-INFLUENZAL ANGINA PECTORIS. REMARKABLE HEART'S-ACTION. RECOVERY.

A lady had suffered off and on for weeks from neuralgia of the left sciatic nerve, which yielded from time to time to various remedies, but never got well. Suddenly one day the pain vanished from the limb and she was struck with intense pain at the heart. Happening to be calling at the very time of the attack I found her in a most perilous condition. She was cold and livid. The pain, which was of a stitching kind, was so intense, that she dared not take a breath, and was gasping when I found her. The heart's action was tumultuous and violent, with an extraordinary sharp clapping sound audible at several feet distant from the patient. She felt she was dying. I gave her a dose of Aconite 3 immediately, and repeated it every minute until she came round, which, happily, she did after one or two doses. But she did not altogether lose the pain, and for weeks was unable to lie on the left side on account of its causing the pain and the most alarming heart's action. Aconite 3 was followed by Camphor (in pilules), and it was after the administration of Camphor that the true nature of the illness declared itself. The state of collapse was followed by symptoms of fever accompanied by intense pains in the back, so characteristic of influenza, and pains in both limbs.

The medicines had relieved the vital organ of the chief incidence of the influenza poison and driven it down to the lower limbs. There it gave an additional proof of its presence by producing an extravasation of blood near the right knee. Haemorrhage and extravasations of blood have been a very frequent manifestation of the influenza poisoning. With the pains there was the intense restlessness so characteristic of Rhus, and Rhus gave great relief. For the complete restoration of the heart to its normal state, many weeks of treatment were required. Carbo vegetabilis, Spigelia, and occasionally Camphor were the chief medicines given.

Chapter 8 ANEURISM.[Aneurism]
THE chief diseases to which blood vessels are liable and degeneration of

their walls with loss of elasticity, and consequent abnormal dilatation. In the veins the condition produced is that known as Varicosis, in the arteries the ultimate result is Aneurism.

In the case of the veins disease is less serious than in the arteries. The internal strain is less severe, and is caused by the downward pressure of the weight of the blood and not by the onward pressure of the heart's contraction. Then there are the valves of the veins to distribute the force of the blood's weight. Rupture of a varicose vein is a comparatively rare occurrence considering the commonness of the affection. With aneurism it is altogether different. The distention goes on increasing steadily unless the disease is checked by treatment, and when the strain can no longer be borne by the diseased walls, rupture inevitably takes place, and unless the rupture is exceedingly minute death immediately follows.

Many cases of what is popularly called "breaking a blood-vessel" are of this kind.

But all arteries that are degenerated do not necessarily give rise to aneurism. The case of Andrew M.(XX.), is one in point. In this case the disease of the artery only led to hypertrophy of the heart. In other cases, as in the arteries of the brain, disease may lead to ruptures of greater or smaller extent without the formation of aneurism. In these cases the rupture gives rise to attacks of apoplexy. Aneurism may form on the arteries within the skull, and when it does it is generally fatal before reaching a large size. The most dangerous places in which an aneurism can form cranial cavity. In these localities the arterial wall is comparatively unsupported and the continued pressure of the heart's contractions soon expands the aneurism to the limits of its distensibility. In the localities where the arterial wall has solid structures to support it in the process of distention, the pressure has to wear them away before it bursts the vessel.

An intra pericardial aneurism-that is, one which springs from that portion of the aorta which is enclosed within the pericardial sac-is, unfortunately, quite impossible to diagnose. It is hardly to be guessed at; as it never reaches a size large enough to be discovered by physical signs.

I will now relate a case in point. The patient was under my care just over a year. She had many symptoms which could not be ascribed to the aneurism and indeed she had a complication of diseases.

CASE XXXIII.-ANEURISM, ETC. RUPTURE WITHIN PERICARDIUM.
Hannah S-, 46, came to my clinic at the Homoeopathic Hospital on the 25th of April, 1885, complaining of the following symptoms :-

Burning pain in chest; tightness and burning pain from under scapulae, up the spine and through each breast, first one and then the other. Has had pain in back for years. Has had a dry hacking cough night and day for two months. Has a headache at the vertex as if she had been felled. Catamenia have ceased for fourteen months; she has flushes and perspirations. Sleeps heavily.

She is very nervous, cries at the least thing. Has much worry.

Tongue white, appetite very bad; for drinks she takes tea and also beer. Is gouty.

Treatment Ignat. 3, four times a day.

(She had a sister die of cancer and she fears it herself. An aunt has severe heart disease. Her mother gave me some additional particulars after death which may be best given here: All her life she was delicate. As a child she suffered much from cough and used to be short of breath. At the age of 21 she was thought to be in a consumption, and a physician who was consulted about her (Dr. Fuller), told her mother to get her away at once to Hastings or the South of France.)

May 9th.-Chest very much better, but

has neuralgia badly. Face flushed. Feels well.

Treatment Argent nit. 5, alternately with Ignatia.

June 6th.-Head much better, but feels very weak. Backs of eyes affected. Tongue quite white in morning. Repeat.

August 29th.-She has been at the seaside. Her head is bad and the pain seems to have affected the eyes, which were much inflamed and red all over last week; now the sight is dim. Has sharp pains in left breast. Has had sixteen abscesses in it in former times.

The pain is sharp, shooting from the region external to the breast to a nodule situated above the centre of the upper edge of the gland, the size of a hemp seed. This nodule is very tender to touch, but it cannot be otherwise distinguished from similar nodules situated along the opposite border. The left breast is very lumpy. She never nursed with her right.

Tongue coated, white as milk in the morning. Bowels confined.

Treatment Bryon. I, four times a day.

September 12th.-Pain and soreness nearly all gone; only a pricking left, not stabbing as before. Eyes rather bad. Repeat.

October 10th.-Her back is very bad since the pain left the chest. It extends up the whole spine and there is ringing in the ears. The mistiness of vision is increased.

Treatment Gelsem. 3, four times a day.

October 24th.-Has had no headache for a fortnight. Has much pain up the spine to the nape. Feels the pain in the left breast now and then; occasionally in the right breast also.

Treatment Conium 3, alternately with Gelsem.

At Christmas she was laid up at home with an attack of pleurisy, and she did not attend at the hospital again until April 14th, 1886, upon which date I find the following note:- Eyes much better. The chest has never quite got over the attack of pleurisy. Has cough in the morning; not much phlegm. Is very short of breath.

Examination. Lungs: Increased vocal resonance and fremitus on right side, no friction.

Heart: First sound accentuated at apex. Action hurried.

Treatment Arsen iod. 3x two grains night and morning. Bryonia I, four times a day.

April 21st.-Was very well till yesterday, when she had several spasms of pain in the left side coming on in the afternoon. She attributed this to the cold winds.

Treatment Iod. 2x, Bryon. I, every two hours alternately,

April 28th.-The pain was better till yesterday, when it came on worse, and to-day it is very bad, She has lost rest and is hysterical. The chest is tender. She becomes much distended. The pain is continuous, burning. Has flushes. Tongue white. Appetite very bad. Has much wind. Bowels confined when she takes milk. Pulse frequent.

The pain does not catch the breath as it did. She does not feel it after being in bed four hours. If she moves her right arm, she feels faint at once and then the pain comes on.

Treatment Acon. 1x, one drop four times a day.

May 5th.-Pain came on badly from 11 o'clock this morning. Before this was very free from it. Bowels confined. Pulse 120. Feels quite well in general health. Always had neuralgia worse in morning.

Treatment Calc. phos. 6x, two grains night and morning. Acon. 1x, four times a day.

May 16th.-Has kept very well up to last night, when the pain was very sharp and left a red spot on the shoulder. Pulse 120.

Treatment Calc. phos. 6x, two grains night and morning. Bryon. 1, four times a day.

May 26th.-Pain very much better. Has had the easiest time since last October. She can turn on her side now. Pulse 116.

She has a good deal of flatulence, with choking in the throat and hysterical symptoms. Tongue white, appetite poor. Repeat.

This was the last day of her life. Early the following morning the patient's son came to me in great agitation to say his mother had been taken suddenly with a fit, that she was quite unconscious, "her face having gone different colours." A quarter of an hour later I was at her house and found her quite dead in the spot where she had fallen. She had taken her breakfast as usual; seemed quite well; had done some household duties and was in the act of making her boy's bed when she fell. Her mother mentioned that a month before she had had a curious sensation at the heart, which compelled her to throw herself on the bed: she felt as she had never felt before.

I will now give my notes of the Autopsy which took place the day after her death.

Body well nourished. Chest resonant. On opening the chest the right lung was found slightly adherent on inner aspect, emphysematous and oedematous, congested at the base, puckered and somewhat fibroid at apex; bronchi filled with sticky mucus. Left lung less emphysematous than right in upper lobe; emphysema in patches, as if recent, in lower lobe; less congested than right and no oedema; a good deal of bronchial congestion.

Heart: Pericardial sac contains a currant-jelly clot weighing about 3 ounces. Heart firmly contracted; valves on right side healthy. Mitral valve slightly thickened. Aorta much diseased; an aneurism about the size of a Tangerine orange (containing scarcely any organised clot), beginning within the pericardium, had opened by a small rupture into the sac. The muscular substance of the heart was soft and fatty.

On opening the abdomen the omentum was found joined by adhesions to the abdominal wall and pelvic viscera. The liver was much adherent to the abdominal wall. The kidneys showed signs of interstitial nephritis, fibrous spots being evident in the substance of the organ and the capsules adhering. The uterus contained a fibroid tumour the size of a walnut: the ovaries were contracted from chronic inflammation.

I have given this case in full to show how serious a disease may exist without giving any definite signs of its presence. Had the aneurism been altogether outside the pericardium, it would have attained a much larger size before rupturing and would probably have reached some spot where its pulsations would have been felt externally. Looking back over the case I am inclined to attribute the persistent pain up the spine to the presence of the aneurism.

The pain complained of on April 21st was undoubtedly due to it and perhaps ought to have made me suspect its presence. But the alleviation of the pain under treatment made the supposition a less likely one; and the presence of other evident morbid conditions in the lungs and elsewhere still further masked the case.

There is another point in the case worth noting, and that is the presence of hysterical symptoms. As is not unfrequently the case, these symptoms, so far from being an indication that the disease was imaginary or nothing of consequence, had their origin in the presence of some grave organic change.

I will now give a case in which the aneurismal tumours were outside the pericardial sac altogether. In this case there was no difficulty about the diagnosis, and the treatment was attended with the best results.
CASE XXXIV.-ANEURISM OF THORACIC AND ABDOMINAL AORTA, WITH VALVULAR DISEASE AND HYPERTROPHY OF THE HEART RELIEVED BY Lycopodium, AND PRACTICALLY CURED BY Baryta carbonica.

The patient was a labourer, 36 years of age. When he first came to me he had been incapacitated from work for sixteen months. He complained chiefly of pains about the chest. There was found to be a large aneurism springing from the arch of the aorta and extending into the right side of the chest, and another, smaller one, from the upper part of the abdominal aorta. There was also extensive valvular disease of the heart, and hypertrophy.

He first received Lyc. 6, two drops three times a day. This was continued for a fortnight. There was improvement in the symptoms at first, but as he then seemed at a standstill I changed the prescription to Bary.-carb. 3x, three grains three times a day. I was led to give this medicine in this form by the success of the late Dr. Torry Anderson in a case reported by him a short time before. I have given the same medicine in higher attenuations, and also Baryta muriatica, in similar cases, but without encouraging success. The prescription was amply justified by the result in this instance. The patient improved steadily, and when he last came to see me, nearly two years later, he was then in full work as a labourer on the railway just as before his illness. He said he felt better than he had done at any time since he was first taken ill; he could see better; the pupils were equal, and responded equally to light. The size of the thoracic tumour, as indicated by percussion, was diminished.

The power of Bary.-carb. over the heart and arteries is suggested by the following symptoms taken from Allen :"Violent long-lasting palpitation." "Palpitation of the heart when lying on the left side." "A fullness in the chest with short breathing, especially on ascending, with stitches in the chest, especially on inspiration." "Dull stitches under the sternum, deep in the chest, followed by a bruised pain at the spot." "Throbbing in the back and severe pulsation during rest." "Great weakness; can scarcely raise herself in bed; if she does, the pulse immediately becomes rapid, jerking, and hard, and after several minutes scarcely perceptible." "In the morning, at 8.0, suddenly feels as if the circulation ceased; a tingling in the whole body extends into the tongue and the ends of the fingers and toes, with anxiety for fifteen minutes; then feels deathly tired."

I will now give particulars of the case in more detail. The sphygmograms show increased resiliency of the arterial walls under treatment.

Jesse F., 36, labourer, short, squarely

built, fair; admitted June 27th, 1884. He complained of pain in the lower part of the chest, and some headache. He had never had rheumatic fever. Fifteen years before he had primary syphilis, but no secondary symptoms. In other respects his health had been good. Four years before he had suffered from giddiness for a month; never giddy since.

About sixteen months before he had pain in the loins and hips on getting up in the morning, and was compelled to give up work in consequence. Two months before admission he felt tightness in both hypochondria, and gnawing and shooting pains; in the epigastrium he had a great pain, as if something were stuck through him. He then went into St. Thomas's Hospital, where he remained five weeks, but received no benefit. He then tried to work, but was compelled to desist as the pain came on again.

When admitted, the pain was just at the level of the nipples. Occasionally it became easier in front and then came on at the back of the chest; it was aggravated by his work, especially when he stooped. He never fainted; did not suffer from headaches. Had always taken food pretty well, but had pain after it. This very often caused him to vomit; a symptom which had been especially troublesome the last two months. The pain made him restless in bed, could not find an easy position; he used to lie best on his right side. He got short of breath when the pain came on, and on exertion. Lately the pain has been worse on the right side, with a numb sensation down the left arm. No difficulty at all in walking. Bowels confined, have been for a long time; has had to take opening medicine. Pulse very collapsing; the arteries can be seen to jump and lengthen out; they are tortuous.

The recoil is very smart and quick. Arteries not well filled during diastole. Left pulse is slightly delayed; very little, but just enough difference to be noticeable.

Physical examination on June 28th

gave the following result :-Cardiac dullness reaches to episternal notch, and bulges to the right side for about one inch. The dullness is not much increased downwards. Apex-beat in nipple line. Expansile pulsation can be felt in episternal notch. Very apparent pulsation in the epigastrium. On palpation there, about three inches below the xiphoid cartilage, and a little to the left side, a pulsating swelling can be felt, and the part is very tender.

In the Mitral Area, systolic and diastolic bruits. Aortic Area: short and rather rough systolic, heard in the vessels of the neck, and a long blowing diastolic, heard all over the dull area and episternal notch, and continued some distance to the left side in the line of the aortic arch. In the Left Auricular Area a systolic bruit is heard. No dullness behind, and no bruit to be made out.

The femoral pulses are equal. No bruit to be made out in them.

The preceding sphygmogram was

taken on this day.

The right pupil is often very large; but it varies a good deal; to-day it is the same size as the left. It reacts to light. He has a cough, but not much expectoration.

When the pain is bad he has some difficulty in breathing. He has been hoarse at times; this comes on irregularly. He loses his voice, so that he can hardly speak. Right back duller than left, breathing feebler, increased vocal resonance and fremitus. Bruit audible all down the spine. The spine is not tender. There is a tender spot about the angle of the left scapula, but nothing abnormal is to be heard there.

Treatment Lycop. 6, two drops three times a day.

I afterwards gave Hydras. 0, gtt. iv. in a wine-glassful of water night and morning, in addition to the Lycop.

July 2nd.-Temp. last night 101.2 degree; this morning 99 degree. Slept better last night. Pain on right side (hypochondrium) and through to back. A little soreness in epigastrium on swallowing. Bowels moved naturally; pupils equal; no hoarseness.

July 3rd.-Feels better. Bowels better, Has pain in epigastrium after swallowing. Pains in right hypochondrium if he lies on that side. No pain when he lies on his back.

July 5th.-No pain at present. Takes food pretty well.

Yesterday he drank water with his dinner, and had a good deal of pain. Pupils equal to-day; yesterday the right was the larger.

July 9th.-Pains not gone, though better than they were. On examining fundus of eye, arteries were seen plainly pulsating. Taking food well.

July 12th.-Had a good deal of pain the last few nights. Pupils still unequal. Taking food very well. Has not much pain when he moves about.

He was now put on Bary.-carb. 3x, gr. iii. ter die, the others being left off.

July 16th.-The pain seems a little better this morning. Is taking food well. Bowels regular.

July 19th.-Has no pain in the day-time; pains come on at night after lying down.

July 26th.-The pains are better. He seems better in every way. Pupil has returned to normal size (after being dilated by atropine for examination). Takes food well.

Exam.-Examination on this day showed comparative dullness above right clavicle. The degree of the dullness radiating from the right sternoclavicular joint is much less, and the extent of it much smaller than it was.

The corresponding part on the left side gives also a rather flat note. There is still pulsation in the episternal notch.

The apex beat is not felt. No pulsation felt in scrobiculus cordis. Mitral area: first sound not quite pure, followed by a loud diastolic bruit. Tricuspid area: first sound, followed by a marked diastolic bruit. Pulmonary area: systolic and diastolic bruits.

Posteriorly.- The right side about the upper and inner angle of the scapula is slightly duller than the left. The breath sounds are not quite so loud as on the left side, and the cardiac bruit is more audible. Otherwise the two sides are alike.

The bruits are audible over the dull area above the right clavicle, and above the dull part; not so loud in the corresponding part of the left chest. The systolic bruit is heard in the carotids.

July 30th.-Still some pain in the right side, low down in the lumbar region, worse when sitting; not felt at all when walking.

The patient went home on the 31st,

and subsequently saw me as out-patient. The improvement had gone on steadily. He continued taking the Bary-carb.

When he visited me on the 2nd of August I took the following sphygmogram:-

On February 20th, 1888, the patient again presented himself at the hospital. He had been at labouring work on the railway ever since June, 1887, and he managed it as well as ever, lifting and carrying heavy weights as this kind of work entailed. The physical signs showed still further improvement, though the cardiac bruits still remained and there was still a little difference in the pupils.

This case I call a practical cure; the patient was restored to his usual health and usefulness. The aneurism had consolidated and contracted, having become firm enough to resist the pressure of the blood stream even under great exertion. The crippled heart valves remained unaltered but the strength of the heart was so far improved that these defects gave rise to no symptoms.

The Baryta carbonica accomplished, tuto et jucunde, the end aimed at by the heroic and dangerous measures of allopathy which generally seriously damage the patient, even when successful. Among them is the insertion of an electric wire within the sac of the aneurism to promote clotting. This has often proved fatal. Another remedy is Iodide of potassium in massive doses. This drug acts specifically on the heart and is used in the homoeopathic form according to its indications by homoeopathists; but even as used by the allopaths it has met with some measure of success. But at what a price! The patient is lowered by the powerful drug to such a degree that very frequently he never recovers the drugging. Another method is reducing the blood-pressure to a minimum degree by means of starvation. The patient is put on "absolute diet"-that is to say just given enough food to keep him in life and no more.

That there is no possibility of routine practice in medicine is shown by the following case in which the medicine which acted so splendidly in the last narrated completely failed. Homoeopathy has no specifics for diseases-only for patients; and the art of it consists in fitting each case with its own remedy.

Another point of comparison between the two will be found in the symptoms of the voice. In the case of Jesse F., as we know, there was hoarseness and loss of voice. As the aneurism improved this symptom disappeared. In the next case it was the alternation in the voice which first attracted attention. The explanation of this is that the increasing aneurismal tumour presses on one or other of the recurrent laryngeal nerves, paralysing its function to a greater or less degree, and so preventing the proper action of the vocal cords.

CASE XXXV.-THORACIC ANEURISM, CAUSING LOSS OF VOICE. ACTION

OF Carbo animalis.

George P., aged 51, a traveller, came to my clinic at the hospital on May 9th, 1888. He complained of his throat, which he said had been bad for six months. Before that he was quite well. Suddenly one night in November, 1887, he was taken with a sharp pain in his chest and two days later he lost his voice. The pains then gradually subsided and he had little inconvenience till the middle of January, 1888, when he began to suffer from pain again- a dull aching "like indigestion." He has been unable to do any work. On the date of his attendance the voice was thin and reedy- almost falsetto.

He had been having treatment for his "voice" before he came, but, naturally enough, got no better. I suspected the cause and asked him to uncover his chest. At the spot where he had complained of pain was an abnormal amount of dullness in the percussion sound, a very slight bulging was apparent, much throbbing could be felt on palpation. Over the tumour a loud blowing murmur was heard. The valvular sounds of the heart were normal.

There remained no doubt as to the nature of the case-it was one of thoracic aneurism.

He seemed fairly well nourished, but had lost much strength since this came on. He could not walk without bringing on pain on pain. His previous health had been very good. For months he had been a total abstainer, but previously he had indulged too freely in alcohol. The minute blood-vessels of the face were marked and prominent, giving the complexion a dark appearance. Tongue whitish; appetite fair; bowels regular and sleep good. He had a very little cough.

Treatment Baryt. carb. 3x, gr. ij. three times a day.

He got no better, but rather worse, so I made him an in-patient.

On admission, June 11th, 1888, the following particulars were ascertained. In his family history the points of importance were that his mother had died of consumption, and one sister had died suddenly from some cause which he did not know.

Other brothers and sisters were alive and healthy. Thirty years before the patient had had some kind of specific disease but had had no secondary symptoms.

The pulse was 60, fairly full, collapsing; there was no difference between right and left. Urine acid, specific gravity 1012, contains no albumen or sugar.

Under Lycopod. 6, and afterwards Ferrum phos. 6x, and still later Calc. fluor. 6x, he made some progress, and after leaving the hospital on August 18th, he was able to undertake some light employment. Later on he left London and I treated him by correspondence.

On October 24th he sent me the

following report. "The pain is severe at times. It is a sharp burning pain, relieved after lying down for an hour. On getting up in the morning it is comparatively well but it comes on again in half-an-hour or so after moving about."

On comparing the symptoms of various medicines, Carbo animalis seemed to me to come nearest with "sharp, burning stitches in chest, and straining and over-lifting easily produce great pulsation of the heart." I gave this medicine in the 500th attenuation (Boericke & Tafel) and there was immediate improvement, both in cessation of pain and in the condition of the voice. On rarely repeated doses of this medicine he kept in wonderfully good health till the following April, a period of nearly six months.

His occupation entailed a good deal of walking which he was able to accomplish without inconvenience.

After that date he began to be troubled with sleeplessness, the pains returned and his voice was not so well. He felt a great strain on his neck when attempting conversation. His voice was very bad and he felt tired and had occasional headache. This state of things continued with fluctuations till the beginning of the following winter when Thuja in high attenuation temporarily checked the downward progress. The winter tried him much and he was laid up with colds. A cough set in which was relieved by Nitric acid; but the lung symptoms again became worse, necessitating medical attendance on the spot and he passed out of my hands. I heard that he died quite quietly not long after. There was no sudden collapse, Death occurred from general failure of strength and not from sudden rupture.

The following case, though incomplete, may be mentioned in this connection. CASE XXXVI.-THORACIC ANEURISM. GREAT IMPROVEMENT FROM Lycopodium AND Baryta carb.

In September, 1894, a gentleman was advised to come from the country to consult me, his allopathic doctors having pronounced him to be suffering from aneurism, and having given him no encouragement as to the future. I was able to confirm their diagnosis, there being a very evident pulsating tumour in the second left interspace, the tumour being the seat of a stitching pain felt up into the left shoulder at times. He also suffered a good deal from difficulty of breathing. But I did not take such a gloomy view of his prospects as his former advisers. I was able to promise him that homoeopathy would, in all probability, give him great relief, and might eventually cure him. The general symptoms pointed to Lycopodium-Loss of flesh, soreness at commissures of lips, tendency to flatulence and constipation, with a little eczema about the anus; urine thick at times; and Lycopodium, given in the 30th potency, promptly relieved him of pain, and did him great good generally. In November last, there being a check in the improvement, he was put on Baryta carb. 3x. Since then I have not seen him, as he lives in the country, and having had a severe cold and an attack of bronchitis, he had been compelled to call in local medical aid. He was, however, able to report in January of this year (1895) that in spite of these trying circumstances his heart had troubled him very little,"in fact, it is better than it has been for some time.

Chapter 9 DIET AND REGIMEN.[Diet and Regimen]

THERE are no more troublesome symptoms in many cases of heart disease than those referred to the digestion. The heart and stomach are very near neighbours. The mid-riff, or diaphragm- the thin muscular wall which divides the cavity of the chest from the abdomen, and plays such an important part in the function of breathing-is the only thing which separates the heart from the stomach. The lower part of the heart rests on the diaphragm, and the upper part of the stomach impinges against the diaphragm's under-side. It follows that when the stomach is over-distended either with food or flatulence, or, which comes to the same thing, when the stomach, by reason of defective dress, is not allowed sufficient room for the discharge of its functions after a meal has been taken, the heart is incommoded and distressed.

But there is even a closer relation between heart and stomach than that of proximity; they are both supplied by the same nerve-the vagus, or pneumogastric-and each organ is thus in sympathy with the other, and apt to feel the effect of any disorder affecting it.

Thus it happens that many persons think they have heart disease when they have nothing worse than indigestion, whilst some who have heart disease find indigestion the most distressing of all their troubles. Several instances of this kind have been recorded in the foregoing pages.

When a damaged heart is fully compensated, and no symptoms are occasioned, the patient may be considered as cured, and no special rules need be laid down; he may eat and live generally, just as ordinary sensible people do. In those cases in which the compensation is incomplete, care will have to be observed in proportion to its defectiveness. In such a case the indulgence of a hearty appetite- a good meal of steak and beer for instance- is quite sufficient to put an end to a patient's life. The best rule is in such a case for the patient to be dieted in exactly the same way as one who suffers from weak digestion. Meals to be taken at regular times; known indigestible or rich foods to be avoided; warm foods to be preferred to cold, and all done up meats to be forbidden. Stewed mutton is the most easily digested of all red meats. When there is much flatulence, soups are undesirable, and generally the quantity of liquids taken should be scrupulously regulated. One most important point should not be overlooked: a patient should never sit down to a meal when tired.

A rest before and after a meal must be the rule. If by any chance the meal-time comes, and finds the patient tired, something very light and warm must be given (such as a cup of scalded milk-cold milk into which boiling water has been poured in equal quantities-or a few tablespoonfuls of strong soup), and the patient must wait until rested before taking the proper meal.

In gouty cases, mutton broth and chicken broth are as a rule preferable to beef tea, when solid meat cannot be taken. A "three-meat-tea" made of mutton, veal and beef is better than beef tea alone. Bread is often a difficulty, and when it is, it should be avoided altogether, and some plain biscuits taken instead. I have known plain hard biscuits with finely grated cold corned beef spread over it make an excellent breakfast in an extreme case of heart weakness. Semi-digested foods, like Benger's Food, are often useful and must be borne in mind.

Of course, this only applies to the period when the heart has not recovered its proper balance. When that result has been brought about the patient may be guided by his sensations, like other people.

There are times when a period of semi-starvation in necessary to a heart's recovery. In a plethoric patient the heart may suddenly find itself, from a variety of causes, unable to deal with the mass of blood in the patient's body.

Tumultuous and irregular action is then the result. In such a case absolute rest, and a diet that is just enough to keep the patient alive, the amount of fluids being reduced to a minimum, will, in a short time, relieve the over-burdened organ, and give it time to recover, and then proper remedies will come in to establish the cure.

The question of alcohol is to be decided by each individual case. Other things being equal, the habitual use of alcohol is undesirable for many reasons. In the first place, as it is such a valuable heart stimulant in emergencies, its effect as a medicine will be seriously discounted in one who takes it regularly. Then, like all special stimulants, its permanent effect is not to strengthen and nourish the stimulated organs, but the reverse. This is seen in the many cases of disease of the heart and arteries traceable to indulgence in alcohol, illustrations of which have been already given. Alcohol is not a nutrient, but on the contrary tends to deprave nutrition. At the same time it may be a question in any case whether the habitual use of a stimulant may be left off with advantage, or whether it will not be the less evil of the two to retain it. This must be left to the judgment of the medical attendant, who will take all the points into consideration.

Coffee and tea enter into the same category as alcohol, and of the two coffee is much the more powerful heart stimulant, and is often in emergencies of the greatest value as a palliative.

The propriety of their use must be judged in each case, but as a general rule their habitual use should be avoided.

REGIMEN.

Closely allied to the question of diet is that of air and exercise.

Air is a prime necessity in heart cases, in some of which "air-hunger" is extreme. The difficulty in our climate in winter is how to get it pure enough, and not too cold. When possible it is desirable to have two rooms on the same landing, entirely at the disposal of a patient. By this means I was able to provide the air necessary in an extreme case of heart suffering throughout one of the severest of recent winters in London. The patient was wheeled from one room to the other, and when one room was unoccupied, a large fire was kept up in it and the window opened; the door was also left open, and also the door of the room occupied by the patient. The windows of the latter room being closed, the air had to pass through the unoccupied room, and was thus warmed before it reached the room where the patient was.

Exercise in some form is as necessary for persons with diseased hearts and blood-vessels, as it is for other people.

The points to determine are, what kind of exercise and how much. In those whose valvular and arterial lesions are fully compensated, any exercise or work that can be performed with comfort may be indulged in. Until that stage has been reached, or when a heart is beginning to fail, walking on the level is the best form of exercise. Stairs are a great difficulty in many cases, and some have found great relief by going upstairs backwards. The limbs have better purchase on the body weight in this method, and there is no bending forward and cramping of the breathing space.

When the heart is very weak, no active exercise at all can be taken. In such cases general massage and passive movements are a great advantage. This secures all the effects of exercise without expense of energy on the part of the patient, without any strain on the heart and without fatigue.

In cases of heart disease in which the stage of possible recovery is passed, it becomes impossible for the patient any longer to lie in bed. The recumbent position places the breathing apparatus at a disadvantage, and gives rise to such a degree of breathlessness that rest or sleep is out of the question. The most comfortable position is sitting in a chair with the legs down, and a rest in front for the head. For a time propping up a patient in bed with pillows may suffice; but before the end the additional relief of letting the limbs hang down is often required.

The consequence of this is, the limbs become dropsical; the dropsy rising higher as the circulation becomes more feeble .

In such cases good nursing is a primary requisite; scrupulous attention to the skin is required to prevent bed- sores. The best means is the application of whiskey dabbed on the most tender parts, which are afterwards powdered.

When there is any soreness, Hypericum oil is of immense utility. The swollen limbs tend to inflame, crack, and exude. Much comfort may be given by keeping the limbs powdered, and bandaged with light, open-wove bandages.

NEWER REMEDIES.[NEWER REMEDIES]
ADONIS VERNALIS.

The best account of this remedy and the next is to be found in Dr. E. M. Hale's "Lectures on Diseases of the Heart." Dr. Hale has done excellent work in collecting information regarding new remedies and defining their place in the Materia Medica.

Adonis vernalis and Convallaria majalis have both been introduced as remedies from Russia, where they are used as heart remedies among the common people. Adonis belongs to the Ranunculaceae. The indications for its use appear to be:- Rapid and feeble action of the heart, dropsy, scanty urine with albumen and casts. Under its action the cardiac contractions increase in force, the pulse becomes less frequent, more regular and full, the urine increases in quantity and albumen and casts disappear.

CONVALLARIA MAJALIS.

This medicine, according to Hale and others, is most indicated when it is necessary to restore the balance of the right side of the heart. It gives great relief in dyspnoea, in cases of emphysema, fibrous and chronic Phthisis, and in the orthopnoea of mitral disease, increasing the flow of urine.

It has little power over dropsy, but in many functional disturbances of the heart it is of great value. A short proving of Convallaria shows that its action on the heart is truly homoeopathic: "Heart's action weak." "When exercising, heart would flutter for about a minute, then the face would get red, and then there was sensation as if the heart stopped beating, and starting again very suddenly, causing a faint feeling." "Pulse full, compressible and intermittent." "Great pain in the heart."

In nervous palpitation arising from mental shock, or disorder in some related organ, as the ovaries, uterus or stomach, it has proved useful. In Russia it is used in cases of hysteria, epileptiform convulsions, etc.

Convallaria causes many respiratory symptoms. "Dyspnoea, caused by sensation as if filling up in abdomen." "Desire to take a deep breath when sitting." "Great dyspnoea, with faintness and palpitation of the heart.' "Great dyspnoea on making the slightest exertion (without cardiac disorder)."

Convallaria, the Lily of the Valley, proves in its action its relationship to Lilium tigrinum and also to Aloe, the Alliums and Squilla in the digestive symptoms it causes; it is a strong purgative and causes much nausea and vomiting in the morning like the morning sickness of pregnancy.

STROPHANTHUS HISPIDUS.

The seeds of this plant are used for making the tincture and extracting the active principle, Strophanthin. it belongs, to the Apocynaceae family and is therefore allied to Apocynum canabinum. It is a native of Central Africa and is used by natives for making an arrow-poison. There have been no provings, but patients in whom the administration of the drug has been pushed, have complained of "Burning in the oesophagus and stomach with loss of appetite and extreme gastric distress, which not rarely rose to vomiting; sometimes there was diarrhoea." It has been used in substantial doses with success in cases of mitral and aortic disease with much dyspnoea and dropsy; it increases the strength of the heart's beats and stimulates the kidneys to action. The indications given by those who have used it are as follows:- Chronic degenerations of the cardiac muscle, with usually a small, frequent and irregular pulse, great difficulty in breathing and oedemas. Nervous palpitation and arrest of breathing.

It sometimes causes a loathing of food, followed by choking and vomiting after eating, sometimes by severe diarrhoea.

I will conclude by relating a case in which it was given, the case being under my care though the medicine was not prescribed by me.
CASE XXXVII.-A Strophanthus CASE. William G., 16, a delicate looking boy, was admitted to the Homoeopathic Hospital on November 25th, 1893. He had had rheumatic fever two years before; and four months before admission rheumatic pains again came on lasting for three months. Up till a month ago he was able to go about and even run up stairs. A week before admission he was taken with cough and shivering, and during the week he had vomited.

On admission he was unable to lie down in bed, had to be propped up in order to breathe; he had a frequent short, dry cough, without pain. The feet, especially the left foot, were swollen, pitting on pressure. The temperature was normal. He had a white tongue; for three days before admission he had been unable to retain any food on his stomach. There was no pain after food but he had much flatulence which he brought up with a great sense of relief.

Examination showed the following condition:

Heart: greatly dilated, pulsation diffused. Loud double bruit in mitral region, with accentuated second sound. In pulmonary and tricuspid areas the second sound is accentuated and reduplicated.

Lungs: loud heart sounds at apices, dullness at both bases and moist rales half way up right lung. Loud heart sound at left base also, but in a smaller area.

Expectoration of bright blood seven days. Cough worse by lying down.

Treatment Strophanthus 0, one drop every four hours was prescribed by the House Physician, Dr. Lambert, to whom I am indebted for the notes of the case.

November 27th.-Swelling of legs nearly gone, cough troublesome through the night. No blood. Bases clearer. Urine alkaline, phosphates, no albumen.

November 29th.-Bases much clearer. No expectoration. No swelling of legs.

December 2nd.-Head aching badly over eyes. Slept badly last night.

December 4th.-Temp. 99.6 degree last evening. Some consolidation still at bases.

December 6th.-Better. Mitral systolic bruit quite disappeared, only the praesystolic heard now. Yesterday had pains in shoulders and burning sensation in feet. Bases of lungs clear, no crepitations.

December 7th.-Temp. 100.2 degree.

December 9th.-Doing well. Slight stiffness in shoulders still.

December 11th.-Temperature rises slightly in evenings. He feels better than he has done for three months.

December 12th.-Praesystolic bruit less harsh. Sounds improved in mitral area. No pain now Stiffness in shoulder.

The Strophanthus was now discontinued and I prescribed Bry. 30 instead.

December 13th.-Shoulder better but neck stiff.

Treatment Act. rac. 30, every two hours.

December 14th.-Back better.

Head left home cured of all acute symptoms on December 20th.

In this case the medicine was eminently homoeopathic, the gastric condition corresponding to the effects of the drug as well as the state of the heart. In this connection it may be mentioned that a case has recently been recorded (see Homoeopathic World of December, 1894), in which

Strophanthus was given to a dipsomaniac, aged 63, for weak heart and intermittent pulse in doses of seven drops, three times a day. After the first dose he was seized with nausea and such a permanent repugnance to alcohol that he stopped stimulants entirely. On this hint Strophanthus was given to other alcoholics with like success-the cure of their craving for stimulants.

Chapter 10 MEDICINES.[Medicines] I NOW come to the last and most important means we possess of counteracting diseases of the heart, or, for that matter, diseases of any kind-I mean the powers of medicines. The popular belief in the power of drugs to cure sick people is ineradicable; and all the efforts of a sceptical Medical Faculty to prove that drugs cannot "cure," and that all the Faculty can do is to "treat" patients, has had no other effect than to cause the lay mind to look to those who have something more encouraging to offer. The popular belief is well founded: the scepticism of the Faculty is the result of a one-sided education which has had the effect of closing its mental vision to all the possibilities that are not dreamed of in the philosophy of the schools.

That drugs will cure has been proved over and over again by millions of experiences, some accidental, some under the guidance of science. The point to be remembered is that drugs do not cure diseases, but patients. I am sometimes asked "Is there any cure for cancer " To which I reply "There is no drug which will cure everybody's cancer; but many cases of cancer have been cured by one or more drugs. Every patient must be treated according to the characteristic features of his particular case, and it is just here that the science and art of medicine come in."

The reason why nearly all the new "cures" that are introduced into old school practice vanish from the old school armamentarium after a very brief career, is not that they are of no curative value, but because those who introduce them regard them as "specifics" for certain "diseases" and have no idea of defining the precise indications for their use. By some lucky chance the first series of patients on whom they try the drug happen to present the proper indications for its use-their cases are in homoeopathic relationship to it, in short,-and they are cured. The allopath knows nothing about this and proceeds to give the same drug to a number of other patients who have the disease called by the same name as that the first patients had, but not presenting the same characteristic indications, and the drug fails to do good. Henceforth it is thrown aside as "unreliable" or "useless," until some despised homoeopathist takes it up and "proves" it, thus finding out what are its characteristic symptoms. Thenceforth it takes its place in the homoeopathic Materia Medica as a valued and trusted implement of the art and science of Healing.

What is curative action Disease, according to the Hahnemannic conception (and I have not yet found a better), is a dynamic or spirit-like change in the left principle of the organism or of any particular organ or tissue.

When the animating principle is in any way hurt, nutrition is not properly carried on. The microscopic elements of the tissues do not undergo their proper transformations, and the whole organ or the whole body is enfeebled. Unless some new agency is brought to bear on the suffering organism, the tendency is for the disease-action to progress from bad to worse. It is here that the specific medication of Hahnemann steps in, and by neutralising the dynamic change in the life-principle, brings back proper nutrition. Then the feeling of well-being and strength comes back. The amount of repair possible depends in each case on the degree to which the degenerative change has gone in the first instance. Where the tissue elements have been destroyed they cannot be restored; but no one can tell in any case how many elements of undeveloped tissue may lie dormant in a damaged organ, ready to be called into life by proper remedial measures, so that it is always the right course to pursue to aim at cure.

The same explanation applies in the case of the cure of tumours. The vital principle, through some change in its operation, produces instead of normal tissues, tissues more lowly organised, with a different life-history from that of the tissues from which they spring. The nutritional changes are different from those of surrounding tissues, and the appearance of new growths or tumours is the result.

But the agency which produce tumours can also remove them, if only the proper specific medicines are administered by which the perverted action will be reversed.

Much of the disputing that has taken place over the proper method of selecting specifics might have been avoided if only the disputants has perceived that in adjusting the sights different focuses may be made use of.

One practitioner, for instance, will use the fine adjustment, taking a minute observation of the symptoms of a patient in great detail and will find a simillimum to cover the picture. Another, working with a lower power, will take a more general view of the case, and select a medicine which he thinks corresponds to this. Both methods have given admirable results, and both have their place in homoeopathy; and it is not at all my intention to dogmatize as to which is the better plan. I have succeeded with each one where the other has failed me.

It has been very truly said that any medicine may be required in any disease, and the case I have recorded in which Crocus played such a brilliant part is an illustration in point. If therefore I am asked, "What medicines are good in cases of heart disease " I must reply, "All the medicines in the Materia Medica."

At the same time it is a very useful work to single out those medicines which have such characteristic action on the heart that they reproduce the features of the majority of the cases met with, and this I now propose to do. It must always be borne in mind, however, that for successful practice it is necessary to take into consideration the whole of a patient's symptoms, more especially the characteristic mental and moral symptoms, in selecting a medicine, and unless the correspondence is good all round only a partial result must be looked for.

The following list may be taken as the selection I should make for my own use if I were limited to a definite number of drugs. Aconite, Ammonium carbonicum, Apocynum, Arnica, Arsenicum album, Arsenicum iodatum, Aurum, Baryta carbonica, Baryta muriatica, Belladonna, Bryonia, Cactus, Calcarea carbonica, Camphora, Carbo animalis, Carbo vegetabilis, Causticum, Cimicifuga, Coffea, Crocus, Crotalus, Digitalis, Gelsemium, Glonoin, Iberis, Ignatia, Iodium, Kali carbonicum, Kali iodidum, Kali muriaticum, Kalmia latifolia, Lachesis, Lilium tigrinum,

Lithium carbonicum, Lycopodium, Lycopus virginicus, Mercurius, Moschus, Naja, Natrum muriaticum, Nux vomica, Phosphorus, Plumbum, Psorinum, Pulsatilla, Rhus toxicodendron, Spongia, Sulphur, Tabacum, Thyroidin, Vanadium, Veratrum album, Veratrum viride. To these may be added three which have been largely used of late in old school practice, Adonis vernalis, Convallaria majalis (the Lily of the Valley), and Strophanthus.

I will now briefly sketch the leading indications for the use of each. Symptoms taken direct from the Materia Medica are in inverted commas.

ACONITE.

Aconite is likely to be called for in all inflammatory affections of the heart (especially those accompanying rheumatic fever), in hypertrophy of the heart, fainting, palpitation and angina pectoris. In all heart disturbances caused by fear, or fright, or anger, Aconite is the first medicine to be thought of. With the Aconite heart there is anxiety and pallor; faintness on sitting up. In the cases where fever is present there in intense restlessness and mental tension; in other cases there is coldness and collapse. In all cases where the characteristic fear of death is present, and especially when the patient is clairvoyant and predicts the time of death, Aconite will do all that is required.

The pulse of Aconite is rather hard, strong and contracted, or else it is feeble.

There are shooting and pricking pains in the chest; great oppression of breathing; sense of anguish in the chest; intense pains in all directions, especially down the left arm, with numbness and tingling.

"Tingling of the fingers of left hand as if going to sleep, with anxiety" is very characteristic of Aconite heart affections. There is relief from lying on the back with the shoulders raised. Suited to plethoric individuals.

AMMONIUM CARBONICUM.

A leading feature of this drug is somnolence, with rattling of large bubbles in the lungs, purplish hue of lips from imperfect oxygenation. Dilatation of heart; crushing weight on sternum when attempting to ascend a height (like Aurum, but the latter has not the somnolence); intense intolerance of a warm room; cough with bloody sputum; palpitation with dyspnoea and retractation of epigastrium; cyanosis. Ammonium carbonicum is a venous medicine and corresponds more to the right heart than the left.

APOCYNUM CANNABINUM.

This drug has been called the "vegetable trochar," on account of its powerful action in removing dropsies by diuresis. The best account of it is to be found in the "Homoeopathic Recorder" for November, 1892, in a lecture by Dr. S.A. Jones.

The chief indications are:-Oppression at the chest; this may be so profound as to make speaking difficult. The most characteristic pulse is a very slow pulse: this is the effect of large doses, but small doses have caused an exceedingly rapid pulse, so either may indicate the drug.

The most characteristic mental symptom is a bewildered state. A number of cases of tobacco poisoning producing heart symptoms and dropsies have been cured with this drug. It belongs to the same natural order as Strophanthus.

Apocynum has been almost exclusively used in the lowest potencies. According to Dr. Jones, watery infusions with just enough spirit to keep them from fermenting are the most efficacious in dropsical cases.

ARNICA.

The chief indications for the use of Arnica will be found in the history of injuries, strains or over-exertion. Heart affections in athletes will require this remedy.

Characteristic symptoms are :-"Bruised pains in the chest, and compression;" "Palpitation;" "Painful pricking in the heart, with fainting fits;' "Cough with expectoration of blood." Most suited to plethoric red-faced persons.

ARSENICUM ALBUM.

"Great oppression at the chest." "Violent and unsupportable throbbing of the heart, chiefly when lying on the back and especially at night." "Irregular action of the heart, sometimes with anguish."

"Shivering or great heat and burning in the chest."

Arsenic is called for in many conditions of weakened or degenerated heart. In order to secure its full action the constitutional indications for the drug must be present, or at least some of them. Great chilliness; desire for warmth; unquenchable thirst for small quantities frequently. Burning pains. Anxiety, restlessness, and excessive anguish which allows no rest, principally in the evening in bed, or in the morning on awaking, and often with trembling, and cold sweats; oppression of the chest; difficulty of breathing, and fainting fits. Unhealthy, dry, scurfy skin. Effects of over-indulgence in alcohol or tobacco.

Many cases of angina pectoris and fatty heart will need this drug. It affects the left heart more especially (Phosphorus the right).

ARSENICUM IODATUM.

As many of the cases narrated in this work were treated with Iodide of Arsenic, it may be well to state here how I first came to use it.

As far as I recollect, it was from observing the marked improvement in the heart symptoms of patients suffering from both pulmonary and cardiac disease, when I had been led to choose the medicine from the lung symptoms alone. Believing that the improvement was due to the direct action of the salt on the heart, and not to its action on the lungs only, I next gave it in cases where the lung symptoms were not such as would call for it, and then I found its action on the heart was just as marked and just as beneficial as in cases of pulmonary and cardiac disease combined.

Our provings of the salt are very scanty, and beyond irregularity of the pulse, noted by one of the provers, there is nothing in the pathogenesis of the Iodide that would lead us to suppose it had great power over the heart. But the clinical experience of its action in cases of lung disease, which proves that it possesses in large measure the combined powers of its two elements, would be a strong a priori argument in its favour as a powerful heart medicine, both Arsenic and Iodide having a very decided action on that organ. My own clinical experience proves that this is the case. It seems to act on the heart muscle,. arresting degeneration and restoring vitality. The coexistence of a chronic cough or chronic lung affection is the chief indication of preference over Arsenicum alb.

The salt in trituration is not very stable. I have used it almost exclusively in the third decimal trituration, but the alcoholic tincture of the same strength is a very active and reliable preparation.

AURUM.

"Great difficulty of breathing at night and on walking in the open air, requiring deep inspirations." "Continuous aching in left side of chest." "Beatings of the heart irregular, or by fits, sometimes with anguish and oppression of the chest." "On any attempt to walk uphill, or on any little exercise, feels as if there were a crushing weight inside the sternum. He feels that if he did not stop walking the blood would burst through the chest."

The mental sphere gives the great indication of Aurum:

Melancholy and inquietude, with desire for death; despair; great anguish inducing a disposition to suicide. Other leading symptoms are : "Giddiness and fainting;" "Great sensitiveness to cold and yet a strong desire to go into the open air, even in bad weather, because it is found to be a relief;" "Aggravation of all symptoms at night from sunset to sunrise."

Aurum is one of the chief antidotes to

Mercury and is called for in cases of over-dosing with that drug; in syphilitic and mercuro-syphilitic cases; in fatty degeneration of the heart and arteries. In patients whose pulses are hard and unyielding from calcareous deposit there is often found the mental condition of Aurum and in such patients it will do excellent work.

BARYTA CARBONICA.

"Difficulty of breathing with sensation of fullness in the chest." "Pains in the chest relieved partly by eructations and partly by external heat." "Fullness and pressive heaviness on the chest, especially when ascending, with stitches, especially on inspiration." "Very violent throbbings of the heart." "Throbbing of the heart excited by lying on the left side, or renewed by thinking of it."

Baryta carbonica has many symptoms of paralysis and degeneration of tissue : "Heaviness of the whole body;" "Necessity to lie down or be seated;" intellectual, nervous and physical weakness. It corresponds to scrofulous and glandular affections. It is a "chilly" medicine and is indicated by the consequences of chill. It is equally applicable to affections of the heart itself and of its vessels, having cured numbers of cases of aneurism.

BARYTA MURIATICA.

The symptoms of Baryta mur. are much like those of Baryta carb. and Baryta acetica and were originally published together in the same schemes. The salts of Muriatic acid have such strong affinity for the heart that it might be expected, a priori, that the cardiac action of the muriate would be more powerful than the carbonate. I cannot give any clearly differentiated symptoms to distinguish between the two. Allen gives under the muriate: "Beating of the heart irregular, pulse scarcely perceptible;" " Pulse rapid, full;" "Pulse soft and irregular;" "Pain in the back."

Hering mentions "palpitation," "dyspnoea," "oppression," "trembling" and "paralytic weakness." It is suited to scrofulous affections and persons subject to catarrh. In some conditions there is relief to breathing by sitting up with the head bent forward. It has cured a number of cases of aneurism.

The mineral water of Llangammarch in Breconshire, Central Wales, contains Baryta mur. in small quantities along with other chlorides, notably Natrum mur. An account of it will be found in the Homoeopathic World, Vol. XXVII (1892), p. 441. It has recently been advocated in the Lancet (November 24th, 1894, et seq.) as a remedy in heart disease and scrofula. Cases of anaemia with gastric catarrh had dilatation of the heart have received remarkable benefit from this water.

BELLADONNA.

A leading feature in the action of this drug is the intensity of the palpitation it causes. It extends from the heart to the minutest blood-vessels and hence arises the appropriateness of Belladonna for a great variety of inflammations in which throbbing pains are marked. "Violent beatings of the heart (which are sometimes felt in the head)." "Palpitation of the heart when ascending." "Great inquietude and beatings in the chest."

"Trembling of the heart with anguish and piercing pain." "Shooting in the chest, sometimes as from knives and chiefly in coughing and yawning." Respirations short, anxious and rapid. Pulse strong and quick, or full and slow, or small and quick, or hard and wiry.

Belladonna conditions are often induced by chill, especially chill after hair-cutting. There is often redness and bloatedness of the face. It acts best in persons of lymphatic or plethoric constitution, especially persons with blue eyes, light hair, fine complexion and delicate skin.

There are very few heart conditions in which Belladonna may not be called for according to the general and local conditions of the drug.
BRYONIA.
For this polychrest to be indicated some of the leading characteristics among the general symptoms of the medicine must be present : Anxiety, inquietude, fear of the future.

Discouragement. Irascibility and passion. Aggravation of all symptoms on movement, better when lying on painful side or painful part; frequent nose-bleed; lips dry, swollen and cracked; indigestion; thickly coated tongue; sense of weight or stone at chest, worse after meals; constipation; disagreeable, vexatious dreams; dreams of transactions of the day; starting with fright on going to sleep and during sleep. Some of these symptoms should be present as well as local conditions :-"Pressive pains in precordial region;" "Stitches; cramp; oppression; tearing stitches in left side of chest from behind forward, better from rest, worse from motion and deep inspirations." "Palpitation; heart beats violently and rapidly."

"Pulse full, hard and rapid."

Bryonia corresponds to many forms of rheumatism and is indicated in many acute inflammatory affections of the heart, and effusion into the pericardium.

CACTUS GRANDIFLORUS.

This powerful heart-medicine, which we owe to the celebrated Dr. Rubini, and the heroic provings of it by himself and his devoted wife (whose health it is to be feared was permanently impaired by her experience) has recently been discovered and appropriated without acknowledgment by allopathic writers. Cactus has one grand key-note symptom distinguishing it from all other drugs. In many cardiac cases there is a painful sense of constriction about the chest or in the heart itself. When a patient complains of a "sensation of constriction in the heart as if an iron band prevented its normal movement," there is no other medicine to be thought of until Cactus has been given. Cactus, however, will cure many cases of heart disease in which this symptom is not present when other symptoms correspond.

Pricking pains (as the prickly nature of the plant might suggest) are almost as characteristic as the constricting pains. "Pricking pins impeding breathing and movement of body; oppression; cannot lie on left side; blue face; pulse quick, throbbing, tense, hard." "Acute pains and stitches in heart." "Very acute pain, and such painful stitches in heart as to cause him to weep and cry out loudly, with obstruction of respiration." "Dull heavy pains in region of heart, worse by external pressure." "Palpitation violent, aggravated by walking and by lying on left side."

"Rapid, short, irregular beats of the heart, on rapid motions, on slow walking, rising from a chair or turning suddenly."

"Slight excitement or deep thought brings on palpitation." "Nervous palpitation increases gradually with the onset of the catamenia." There is irregular and intermittent movement of the heart. Pulse hard and sudden without being frequent. The heart symptoms often compelled the prover to stand still when commencing to walk and to inspire deeply several times. One peculiar symptom experienced was a "sensation of very annoying movement, from before backward in the cardiac region, as if a reptile were moving about in the interior; worse by day than by night." The usual time of aggravation of the "Night-blooming cereus" is the evening and night.

A tendency to haemorrhages is a distinguishing feature of Cactus grand.

The other members of the Cactus family are potent heart remedies, notably **CEREUS BONPLANDII**, which has among other symptoms the following: "Sensation of a great stone laid on the heart; soon after, sensation as if the chest was broken out just in front of the heart." "Feeling as if the heart was transfixed with a blunt instrument like a bolt." "Slight pricking pain at the heart."

CALCAREA CARBONICA.
One of the leading antipsoric medicines, corresponding to many forms of rheumatism, Calcarea cannot be left out of sight in a catalogue of heart remedies. Its systemic symptoms will be the best guide to its use : "Apprehension, fearing consumption

and heart disease." "Ill-humour, obstinacy, and disposition to take everything in bad part." Obesity or emaciation. Great chilliness, sensitiveness to open air; coldness and clamminess of hands and feet, feeling as if stockings were damp. Cold sweat of head and chest. Acidity, heartburn, hunger soon after eating. Menses too early, and too profuse. Stiffness of limbs; painful swellings of joints and nodosities on fingers and toes.

In the chest we have "Shortness of breath chiefly an ascending." "Wheezing respiration." "Anxious oppression." "Burning." "Palpitation of the heart, also at night, and after a meal, sometimes with anxiety and trembling movement."

heart." "Want of strength and dejection, worse in morning early." "Fainting, especially in the evening, with obscuration of the eyes, sweat on face, and cold in the body, worse on walking in open air." Sensitiveness to strains, like Baryta carb.

There are no conditions of heart and arterial disease that will not be benefited by Calcarea if the above symptoms or several of them are prominent.

CAMPHORA.

In all kinds of spasmodic affections with coldness of the surface and collapse, especially if there is at the same time intolerance of external heat, Camphora is to be thought of. Among the special heart symptoms are found: great anxiety in precordial region; spasmodic stitches in region of heart with oppression of chest when lying on left side, better when turning on right side. Palpitation. Pulse full or weak and imperceptible.

CARBO ANIMALIS.

Carbo animalis has a special relation to the effects of strains, and it also corresponds to many manifestations of secondary and tertiary syphilis. On both these accounts it is brought into relation with diseases of the arteries and aneurism in which strain is a great causative element, syphilis being frequently the original cause of the arterial defect.

In one of my patients it did excellent service for a long time given on the indication: "Sharp burning pains in the chest coming on after moving about, relieved completely by lying down." The symptoms noted under Carbo an. are are "Sharp burning stitches in chest." and "Straining and over lifting produce great pulsation of the heart." A coppery acneous eruption on the face is a further indication. **CARBO VEGETABILIS.** "Tight chest with fullness and anxiety." "Burning pains in region of heart, with congestion in chest and violent palpitation of heart." "Stitches through region of heart and spleen." "Pulse threadlike, weak and faint." "Cheyne-Stokes respiration."

The Carbo veg. Patient must have air; wants to be fanned and to have the room cool. With the heart symptoms there is flatulent indigestion. "All food disagrees, even the most innocent." There is often great and long-lasting hoarseness. Brown-yellow blotches on chest.

CAUSTICUM.

In the case of a young girl recently admitted to the homoeopathic Hospital suffering from rheumatism, with both endocarditis and pericarditis with large effusion, apparently well indicated remedies had little effect.

Pneumonia and pleurisy were added to her other troubles, and incontinence of faeces and urine. This last symptom led me to think of Causticum, especially as it was observed that the cough caused expulsion of urine. Causticum 30 was given, with immediate and rapid improvement in all the symptoms. The effusion was quickly absorbed, and the patient was soon convalescent. A mitral heart symptoms of Causticum are : "Oppression at heart with lowness of spirits; cardiac anxiety." "Stitches in cardiac region." "Burning in region of heart with palpitation." "Palpitation with languor." "Chronic disease of heart in young girls occasioned by overlifting." "Pulse excited towards evening with orgasm of blood."

CIMICIFUGA.

Cimicifuga racemosa, or Actaea racemosa as it is also called, is an important rheumatic an neuralgic remedy, and hence it is often called for in cases of deranged heart. The special heart symptoms are as follows: "Palpitation from the least motion." "Pains from region of heart all over the chest and down left arm, which feels numb and as it bound to the side; palpitation; unconsciousness; cerebral congestion; face livid; dyspnoea; cold sweat on head, and numbness of body."

"Heart's action ceases suddenly; impending suffocation."

Excessive muscular soreness; pains in the nape of the neck; restlessness; twitchings and tremblings; mental gloom and fear of death. "Sensation as if heavy black cloud settled all over him. enveloping him so that all was darkness and confusion, while at the same time it weighed like lead on his head." "Waving sensation in the brain"- all these are additional indications for Cimicifuga.

COFFEA CRUDA.

Excessive sensitiveness and excitability is the leading note of the Coffea condition. All pains are unendurable. It causes violent irregular palpitation with trembling of the limbs. Palpitation after excessive exaltation, joy, surprise. Palpitation with nervous excitement and sleeplessness. Black Coffee (Coffea tosta) is a very valuable heart stimulant under certain conditions of heart failure: palpitation with vertigo and fainting; palpitation from irritable heart; collapse with feeble, frequent pulse.

CROCUS.

I need not add much to what I have said of this medicine in the body of the work apropos of Case IX. It has a "sensation of emptiness in precordial region; stitches beneath heart, worse on inspiration; palpitation and anxiety with sensation of weakness extending from heart through whole abdomen and down to soles of feet."

But for Crocus to cure, the peculiar mental conditions ought to be present: uncontrollable laughter, or else violent alternations of disposition; and the keynote symptom-sensation as if something alive inside, or jumping sensation. Cactus has something like this.

CROTALUS.

Like all the serpent poisons, Crotalus profoundly affects the heart, depressing it's action even to fatal syncope. The most characteristic symptom of Crotalus is a sensation as if the heart was tumbling about or tumbling over and over like a tumbler pigeon.

DIGITALIS.

It would be difficult to estimate the number of lives that have been sacrificed in old-school practice to this potent drug; which is invaluable if properly used and deadly when abused. Its dangers are so great when given in the massive doses of the allopaths that the efforts of their therapeutists are largely directed to finding "substitutes for Digitalis." There are no "substitutes" for Digitalis, for its action is characteristic and unique, and in homoeopathic form it is as innocent as it is powerful.

Other heart-poisons may be discovered, but they cannot take the place of Digitalis.

I remember in my student days Dr. George Balfour, of Edinburgh, pointing out in patients under the influence of Digitalis, that as soon as the pulse became accelerated and irregular on the patient rising from the recumbent to the sitting position the drug ought to be suspended. This is a characteristic feature of Digitalis: aggravation on changing position, and especially on rising from the horizontal. In many a patient has fatal syncope occurred when less careful prescribers have failed to stop the drug in time. For one feature of Digitalis is its "cumulative" effect; that is, the effects of repeated doses accumulate in the system, and sudden symptoms of poisoning appear, as if all had been given in one large dose.

The condition of heart which calls for Digitalis is a weakened heart, or a dilated heart. Among the symptoms that indicate it are irregular, feeble, rapid action, on any exertion, ad rising up from the recumbent position. "Faintness on sitting up." "Sudden sensation as though the heart stood still, with great anxiety and necessity for holding the breath." "Feels as if the heart would stop if he dared to move." (Gelsem. has the opposite of this-"feels as if the heart would stop if he ceased to move"). "Angina pectoris; tearing pains in left side of chest and left border of sternum, extending to nape of and shoulders; great anxiety and fear of death; slow pulse."

"Angina brought on by any careless, quick movement; pain extending down left arm." "Pulse and breathing slow, intermittent; irregular, small.

Among the other symptoms of Digitalis are-"Weakness of memory; difficult thinking; anxiety; low spirits; desire to be alone." "Pallor of face, especially on rising from recumbent position." "Faintness and sinking at the stomach, as if he would die." "Soreness and hardness in the region of the liver.

White stools." In the male there is "weakness and erethism of the genital system with spermatorrhoea and great weakness. "Heaviness and paralytic weakness of left arm." "Fingers go to sleep easily; coldness of limbs." "Cyanosis."

GELSEMIUM.

"Pain in heart when rising from a seat." "Effects of grief- oppression and palpitation, worse when thinking of it or spoken to of his loss; sensation of soreness about the heart." "Irregular action; palpitation; hysterical palpitation." "Slow, feeble action of heart" pulse can hardly be felt." "Fear that unless constantly moving her heart will cease beating; with fear of death." "Pulse frequent soft, weak, almost imperceptible; slow pulse." "Hands and feet cold."

The key-note symptom of Glonoin (or Nitro glycerine), as might be anticipated from the nature of the substance, is a sensation of bursting, and throbbing as if about to burst. In the heart itself there is a sense of fullness. "Blood seems to rush to heart and mount rapidly to head." "Violent action of heart, distinct pulsation over whole body." "Palpitation with throbbing, bursting headache." "Sharp pains in heart." "Laborious action of heart; oppression; frequent pulse." "Sensation of fullness and heaviness with laboured breathing." "Severe stitches in heart, extending into back between shoulders." "Patient must have head high; worse lying on the left side; better lying on right."

Glonoin has a prominent has a prominent place in climacteric flushings.

IBERIS.

Palpitation plainly visible over whole chest; worse by walking; better sitting still, but renewed by slightest exertion. Stabbing pains in heart, with constriction in throat. Palpitation with vertigo and choking after walking. Much pain over base of heart, with dull, heavy pain in left arm, and tingling and numbness in finger tips. Weight and pressure in region of heart with occasional sharp, stinging pains, passing from before backward.

Hypertrophy of heart.
IGNATIA.
"Anxious feeling in precordia." "Mental agitation and nervousness accompanying heart affections." "Constriction at heart, with anxiety and disposition to cry." "Palpitation at night and in morning in bed." "Palpitation on the least worry or excitement, or from grief." Ignatia when indicated by local or general symptoms is of the greatest service, both in organic and functional disorders of the heart.
IODIUM.
This medicine is called for in cases of hypertrophy and over-action of the heart, whether occasioned by valvular disease; or not; also in aneurism and diseases of blood vessels, and exophthalmic goitre. There is palpitation, especially after exertion. There is a sensation as if the heart was being squeezed with an iron band. A sense of "goneness" or excessive weakness at the chest and in the heart. Precordial anxiety; constant, heavy, oppressive pain in region of heart. Pulse-accelerated by every exertion; large, hard and frequent; rapid, but

weak and thread-like; small, but very quick and irregular.

Iodium causes extreme emaciation with canine hunger; or, entire loss of appetite; excessive excitability; intolerance of warmth. It is more especially suitable to persons with dark hair and eyes.

KALI CARBONICUM.

Stitching pains are very characteristic of Kali carb., and these are found in the heart as elsewhere; "Stitches about heart and through to scapula." But Kali carb. has a peculiar sensation which is quite characteristic: "Pinching or cramping pains in or by the heart, as if the heart were hanging by tightly drawn cords." Aggravation from 2 to 5 a.m.

KALI IODATUM.

This is another drug which is frightfully abused by the old school. It is one of the most profoundly action agents in the Materia Medica. There is nothing that will reduce weight and strength beyond the point of possible recovery more surely than Iodide of potassium. It is regarded as an anti-syphilitic almost entirely, and is used as a means of diagnosis. Whenever syphilis is suspected, Iodide of potassium is prescribed; if it cures, it is considered that syphilis was present, and if it kills, it is concluded that it was not syphilis. Mr. Jonathan Hutchinson has put on record one of the many cases of this kind. An unfortunate man was admitted to hospital suffering from a skin affection, which was diagnosed as syphilitic, though the patient strongly denied ever having had a primary sore. Iodide of potassium was given, and as the man got worse it was concluded that the dose was not strong enough; thereupon it was largely increased.

The patient then became much worse, purple tumours somewhat like syphilitic nodes appeared in all parts of his body. It was then discovered that these tumours were caused by the drug, which was then suspended. But it was too late-the patient died of the "scientific." treatment to which he had been subjected.

A case of a somewhat different kind

came under my notice a short time ago.

A gentleman;, aged 74, who had had robust health all his life till the last two years, and who looked, except for his appearance of illness, much younger than his age, consulted me recently about his digestion. His history was this. Some two years before, he began to be troubled with an eruption, which appeared in patches about arms and body, and he put himself under the care of a well-known homoeopath. The skin did not get well, though his general health remained excellent. By the advice of a relative, an old school practitioner, he consulted a well-known syphilographer, who at once and unhesitatingly pronounced his disease to be syphilitic. In this case also the patient denied ever having had a primary sore. Iodide of potassium was ordered, and in doses so massive that the medical relative was alarmed, and refused to allow the full amount to be taken. Sufficient, however, was taken to produce the profoundest depression and lowering.

The old man cried like a child without knowing why. And besides this, his digestion, which had been excellent before, was never good after. But-the skin affection disappeared in a fortnight, and the patient congratulated himself on his "cure"

When he came into my consulting room he was plainly a broken man; there was a dusky, drawn, anxious look about him; his weight had dropped from ten stone to little over nine. He could eat very little without distress and a full sensation; attacks of palpitation came on at all times and kept him awake at night. His hands trembled, so that he could not write his usual steady hand. His pulse was extremely frequent, and very small. Here is a sphygmogram I took from his right radial with a pressure of 3 1/2. The valve sounds were clear and no bruit could be detected. His heart had been declared sound by several eminent practitioners, and so it was so far as auscultation could tell; but auscultation cannot discern the Iodide of potassium disease.

I saw him several times within the week. On one occasion I found the pulse normal in force and rhythm, and I then indulged the hope that the condition might turn out to be functional only and transient.

The next day I found the pulse irregular and intermittent or very frequent. The patient (who was unmarried) wished to go to stay with some relatives, and I thought this was the best thing he could do. I have since heard that he died not long after leaving town. He died of-Iodide of potassium.

I cannot be denied that in some cases large doses of Iodide of potassium do seem to benefit, and in some cases of aneurism encouraging success has attended the treatment. My own impression is that, when good result, it is in the cases where there is a strong element of active syphilis at work; the one poison seems to antidote the other. Where there is no syphilis or only a very slight amount, massive doses of

Kali iod. produce irremediable mischief.

Here are symptoms from the pathogenesis which it will be seen correspond pretty closely to those of my patient :- "Fluttering on awaking, giddy; must get up, fearing otherwise that he will smother." "Fluttering of heart and nervousness; feels very weak." "Palpitation, worse while walking." "Darting pains in heart when walking, after abuse of Mercury; after repeated endocarditis." "Pulse accelerated." Profound adynamia will be a leading indication for the use of the drug.

Kali iod. is useful in cases which have been treated with Mercury. In aneurism it has a specific effect, though it is mainly given with the notion of lowering the patient's strength, and especially the blood pressure, so as to give the blood in the aneurismal sac an opportunity of clotting.

KALI MURIATICUM.

The salts of muriatic acid have a powerful action on the heart, and Kali mur. is no exception. It is one of Schussler's remedies, and he recommends it for that condition of the blood which favours embolus; in the exudative stage of inflammatory affections of the heart; in palpitation from excessive flow of blood to the heart; and in hypertrophy. The symptoms which call for it are: "Palpitation with constriction of the chest." "Perceptible, but not accelerated beating of the heart, with coldness in cardiac region." "Pulse accelerated, or soft and sluggish." A white coated tongue is an indication for Kali mur., which is very analogous to Bryonia in its action.

KALMIA LATIFOLIA.

Kalmia Latifolia belongs to the Ericaceae like Ledum and Rhododendron. Like Ledum, its pains travel from below upward, and it is therefore suitable for rheumatic affections which leave the limbs and attack the heart. The pains are sharp and take away the breath.

Pains shoot down into abdomen and stomach. The pulse is slow. With the heart symptoms there is numbness of the left arm. Numbness of parts after pain has left. Pains move from place to place.

LACHESIS.

"Vertigo and fainting from heart weakness"; "palpitation and fainting." "Trembling." "Palpitation with a feeling of constriction, as if the heart were tightly held with cords." "Sense of oppression with cold feet; as the feet get warm the oppression is relieved." "Flushings, throbbings, cold feet, chilblains." "Heart feels as if too large for the chest." "Palpitation with numbness of arm, choking from slightest exertion; relieved by sitting down or lying on right side." The conditions are all-important in Lachesis. Worse after sleep; worse on closing eyes; intolerance of slightest constriction in any part; intolerance of touch; worse when a discharge fails to appear and better when it does appear. This points to its use in climacteric sufferings.

Irritability of temper is an indication for Lachesis.

LILIUM TIGRINUM.

The characteristic sensation of Lilium is somewhat like that of Cactus, a sensation as if the heart was grasped, but there is a difference.

The "iron band" sensation of Cactus is not present with Lilium, nor is the constriction of the latter so enduring.

"Sensation as if heart was grasped, or squeezed in a vice; as if blood had all gone to heart, producing a feeling as if he must bend double : inability to walk straight." "Heart as if violently grasped, then suddenly released, alternately." "Constrictive pain about heart through to scapula." "Sharp pain extending from left nipple through chest to back," indicates Lilium in many heart conditions. "Sensation as if heart was overloaded with blood and it would be a relief to bring up some." "Frequent sensation as if heart stopped, followed by rush of blood to heart and palpitation." "Pain, dull pressure and fullness, with feeling of coldness about the heart." "Heaviness." "Irritability." "Fluttering and faint feeling."

"Conscious pulsations over whole body."

The symptoms are worse by eating ever so little; worse lying on either side; better sitting still.

The mental symptoms of Lilium are characterised by a sensation of hurry combined with a feeling of importance. Like other drugs which cause venous engorgement, it has amelioration in open air and taste of blood in the mouth, also scanty menses. There is a tendency to prolapsus uteri with bearing down or dragging down.

LITHIUM CARBONICUM.

The chief feature of the Lithium heart symptoms is the concomitance of symptoms of the urinary system. "Pressing in region of heart on rising to urinate, better after urinating." Pains in heart before and at time of urinating; also before and at time of menses." "Rheumatic soreness about heart, worse on stooping; pains in limbs; finger joints tender and painful; sleeplessness." "Violent pain in region of heart as she bent over the bed;

morning after rising."

Lithium has proved of great service in valvular affections of the heart, and the condition left after acute inflammation. A concomitant of the heart symptom is "On inspiring, air feels cold even into the lungs."

LYCOPODIUM.

It is more in the general symptoms of Lycopodium than in the special heart symptoms that the indications for its employment will be found.

"Sadness and apprehensiveness, weeps all day, cannot calm herself; sensitiveness, weeps when thanked; irritable, peevish, misanthropic; omits words and letters when writing, uses wrong words; headache, better by uncovering; sinking sensation at pit of stomach, worse in afternoon; fullness after the least food; excessive flatulence; constipation; red sand in urine; burning as from hot coals between scapulae, aggravation of all symptoms in afternoon from 4 to 6 or 4 to 8 p.m.."-These are the leading features of the Lycopodium patient, and some of them, should be present in cases for which it is prescribed.

I will now give some of the special symptoms:-

"Palpitation especially during digestion, and in bed in the evening, sometimes with anxiety and trembling." "Lancinations in the chest, especially the left side." "Sensation as if the circulation stood still." "Pulsating tearing in region of heart."

In all kinds of weakened heart Lycopodium may find a place, and in aneurism and diseases of the arteries. In the last stages of heart disease when the lungs become secondarily engorged, it often renders great help. Iodine and Lycopodium are complementary medicines.

LYCOPUS VIRGINICUS.

This medicine has proved of service in many forms of heart disease-valvular affections, hypertrophy, exophthalmos and aneurism. There is irritability and erethism of the heart with debility. The patient is nervous and irritable, extremities cold. Cough with haemoptysis in connection with heart affections. Palpitation and heart distress, worse morning and evening and when thinking of it. Heart's action tumultuous and forcible, can be heard several feet from the bed. Laboured action. Heart beats slow and weak. **MERCURIUS.**

In the days when it was the fashion to put everybody who was unfortunate enough to enter a hospital under the influence of Mercury, it was no uncommon thing to have patients drop dead from heart failure when simply walking across a hospital ward. Thus Mercury, like its dynamic antidotes, Iodine, Kali iod., Carbo vegetabilis, Lachesis and Belladonna, finds a place in the treatment of states of weakened and degenerated heart. It is no less appropriate when the weakness is occasioned by acute inflammatory states-endocarditis, pericarditis, with or without effusion, and especially when the inflammation is rheumatic in nature.

The leading indications for Mercurius in

general are aggravation at night: profuse sweat which does not relieve, and is offensive in smell; tremor; sensitive to atmospheric changes, worse from both cold and heat; worse in damp weather. Tongue large and flabby, indented by the teeth; white coat; offensive breath. Blood-streaked purulent discharges are a strong indication for Mercurius.

The special heart symptoms are:-

"Weakness at heart as if dying." "Awakens with trembling at heart and agitation as if frightened." "Aching pain at apex of heart, extending upwards towards base; cardiac oppression.' "Palpitation with fear; worse at night; on slightest exertion; with cough and bloody expectoration."

"Pulse full and accelerated, with erethism, frequent at night, slower by day; when slow, weak and trembling."
MOSCHUS.
Musk corresponds very closely to the cataleptic state and hence to fainting fits in all degrees whether there is

organic change in the heart or not. "Weakness to the extent of fainting, with nocturnal coldness of the skin generally." "Fainting fits especially at night, in evening, or in the open-air." "Anxious palpitation." "Apprehension of death and excessive timidity about dying." "Sensation of coldness mostly in the spine with drawing pain." "The air seems cold; the patient seeks the fire-side." "Great susceptibility to the open-air."

NAJA.

In angina pectoris, valvular disease, threatened paralysis from diphtheria, hypertrophy, and effects of grief, Naja takes an important place. Disorders of other organs in which the heart is affected sympathetically, as palpitation accompanying ovarian affections. "Depression and lowness about the heart." "Sensation as though a hot iron had been run into heart and a hundred-weight put upon it." "Inability to speak, with choking, nervous, chronic palpitation." "Severe pains in left temple, cardiac and ovarian regions."

"Sensation as if heart and ovary were

drawn together." "Pains about heart extending to nape of neck, left shoulder and arm, with anxiety and fear of death." Pulse slow, irregular in rhythm and force. Symptoms worse at night; walking; lying on left side.

NATRUM MURIATICUM.

My attention was first was first markedly drawn to the power of Nat. mur. as a cardiac medicine by the signal relief it gave many years ago to a patient, an elderly woman, suffering from extreme hypertrophy due to valvular disease, to whom I had given it principally to relieve constipation. She said nothing had given so much relief to her heart symptoms before. Nat mur. has in its pathogenesis:-

"Anxious and violent palpitation of the heart at every movement of the body, but principally when lying on the left side." "Irregular and intermittent palpitation." "Jerking movement of the heart." Palpitation and intermittent of accelerated pulse after a meal." "Jerking and shooting pain in the region of the heart.

Nat mur. is the "chronic" of Ignatia, and it corresponds to many so-called hysterical conditions. There is melancholy with much sadness and inclination to weep, and the patient is made worse by any attempt to give consolation. The bad effects of a disappointment.

Consequences of self abuse. Results of intermittent fevers in which quinine has been given to excess. The symptoms are worse when lying down, especially at night and in the morning; better from rising up in bed; worse after sleep. The sleep is agitated, dreams of robbers, murders, fire, etc. **NUX VOMICA.**
"Pulsation in the chest and side." "Shootings and blows in the region of the heart." "Palpitation, worse principally after dinner; when lying down; or in the morning; accompanied by nausea, inclination to vomit, and sensation of heaviness in the chest."

Nux, being one of the polychrest medicines, may at any time be indicated in a cardiac case. The above are the chief symptoms occurring in the heart itself, but the following chest symptoms strongly indicate its use:-

"Asthmatic constriction and oppression, worse at night or in the morning, or in bed in the evening; when lying down; when going up an ascent; when walking; after dinner; often accompanied by a choking anxiety; pressure in the epigastrium; humming in the ears; quick pulse, and sweat." "Slow, wheezing respiration." "Tensive pressure in chest as from a weight, principally at night and in the open air."

The sensitiveness, irritability and chilliness of Nux, sensitiveness to open air, sour smelling breath, constipation, early waking (3 a.m.) and falling asleep just when it is time to rise-must all be taken into consideration in prescribing this medicine.
PHOSPHORUS.
"Obstructed respiration and oppression of the chest of various kinds; especially in the morning or evening; also during movement." "Anguish in the chest."

"Heaviness, fullness and tension in the chest." "Lancinations in chest, particularly left side, sometimes prolonged or else when the parts are touched." "Burning pain as from excoriation." "Palpitation:-after a meal; morning and evening; when seated; after all kinds of mental excitement." "Pulse quick and hard." "Fainting fits." "Ebullition and congestion of blood, sometimes with pulsation throughout the body."

The typical Phosphorus patient is dark, tall, narrow-chested and stooping, phthisical and inclined to haemorrhage. Sufferings from chill and from anger call for it; pain in the limbs on change of weather; worse in open air especially when cold; worse morning; evening; in bed; after dinner; some symptoms appear at the beginning of a meal and disappear after it. A characteristic aggravation of Phos. is from lying on left side.

Another is worse from warm food and drink-a drink of cold water will remain in the stomach until it becomes warm and then it is vomited. Among the mental symptoms are- "Hypochondriacal sadness." "Great irascibility, anger, passion, and violence." "Shamelessness." "State of clairvoyance." There is amelioration after sleep. Sleep is disturbed by anxious, distressing dreams, frightful and horrible. Somnambulism.

Phosphorus causes fatty degeneration of all tissues, and many of its symptoms point to its applicability to forms of fatty heart and degenerated arteries; and also to venous stagnations. It corresponds more to affections of the right or venous side of the heart, Arsenicum more to the left.
PLUMBUM.
In cases of lead poisoning there is not unfrequently seen, in addition to paralytic symptoms, profound alteration of the arterial system and heart. In one case which came under my own notice, there were numerous aneurisms principally affecting the lower extremities. Lead sets up granular degeneration of the kidneys and the condition of hypertrophy of the

heart which always accompanies this. It also produces hypertrophy and degeneration of the heart muscle independently. The special heart symptoms of Plumbum are "Violent spasmodic palpitation with anxiety at the heart."

"Pressure on the chest with difficult breathing." Pulse "small; slow; contracted"; or, it may be rapid.

The mental symptoms of Plumbum are "Melancholy"; "Gloom"; "Anxiety"; and "Mental torpor." The great characteristic of the drug is obstinate constipation, stool in the form of balls, abdomen hard, muscles knotted, sense of constriction navel and anus violently retracted.

PSORINUM.

The distinguishing feature of Psorinum is to be found in the condition "better from lying down." Almost all conditions of weakened heart and distressed breathing are better by propping up. When chest symptoms are better lying down, Psorinum will in all probability cure; though Psorinum must not necessarily be excluded in a case if the reverse, "inability to lie down," is present.

"Pain in heart better when lying down, thinks the stitches will kill him if they continue." "Gurgling in the heart, more particularly when lying." "Palpitation: with anxiety, mental disquietude; dislike for work; from coughing; from liver disorders." "Dyspnoea : with palpitation; with pain in cardiac region.'

The intense prostration of Psorinum, with desire to lie down; chilliness, even in hot weather wanting to be wrapped in furs; sensitiveness to stormy weather; irritable, unhealthy skin; fetid sweat and evacuations, will be sufficient to indicate the place of this remedy.

It is closely allied to Sulphur, which it follows well.
PULSATILLA.
The Pulsatilla type of patient is the opposite of that of Nux: Fair haired, fair eyed, inclined to stoutness; mildness

and gentleness of disposition, easily moved to tears or laughter. Pulsatilla is indicated by shifting pains, passing rapidly from one part to another, worse when at rest, when seated, on rising after being long seated, when lying on the side (especially the left,) in the evening before midnight, in a warm room. Better in open air, walking about slowly.

"Shootings in the chest and sides principally at night and when lying down." "Fits of suffocation: worse in evening, after a meal; at night; when lying down." "Congestion of blood in the chest and heart especially at night." "Frequent and violent palpitation, principally after dinner, after moral emotions, provoked by conversation, and often with anguish, clouded sight, impeded respiration, especially when lying on left side." "Anxiety, nervousness, pressure, and burning sensation in the heart." "Numbness, particularly about the elbow very frequently with hypertrophy or dilatation of right ventricle"(Farrington).

RHUS TOXICODENDRON.

This is one of the great rheumatic remedies, the characteristic feature of its pains being relief from motion. There may be aggravation on commencing motion but after the first movement further movement gives relief. (Bry. "The more he moves the worse the pains are.") As soon as the patient remains quiet the pains get worse, compelling him to move again. There is shivering and coldness in the Rhus patient, better from warmth, worse from damp air or from getting wet. Complaints after a wetting, worse at night. Anxious sadness and excessive anguish, especially in evening and at night; desire for solitude and inclination to weep; sleep disturbed by frightful dreams of fire; dreams of the business of the day.

"Weakness in the chest, speech difficult after a moderate walk in the open air." "Shootings and lancinations in the chest and sides of the chest, especially when sitting with the body bent forward; speaking; breathing deeply; seldom when walking or using vigorous exertion." "Tingling in the chest.' "Weakness and sensation of trembling at the heart." "Violent palpitation whilst sitting quietly.' "Shootings in the region of the heart, with painful sensation of paralysis and torpor of left arm." "Transient coldness in the back."

The pulse is full and strong; accelerated and weak; irregular or intermittent.

Numbness of left arm accompanying heart affections is found in Rhus, Acon., Puls., and Kalmia.
SPIGELIA.
Spigelia anthelmia is in the very first rank of cardiac medicines and may be called for in any kind of disorder of both heart and vessels, but as it has been fully dealt with in foregoing chapters (especially pp. 88 to 100) little need be added here. Spigelia is eminently a neuralgic medicine with a preference for the left side. Tearing and stitches in the chest. "Cutting piercing pain through left chest near sternum from front to back."

"Lacerating with constriction." "Dull stitches in region of apex beat." "Dull sticking and pinching from beneath left nipple to region of scapula and upper arm." The palpitation is violent, sometimes audible, with great anxiety and breathlessness. The symptoms are worse: on sitting down; sitting down after rising from bed; bending forward; raising the arms; taking deep inspirations; exertion. Better: from lying on right side with trunk raised. Accompaniments: excessive sensitiveness and weakness; sensitiveness to cold.
SPONGIA.
"Spasmodic constrictive pains in whole chest." "Fullness and obstruction." "Cannot lie with head low without bringing on a fit of suffocation."

"Frequently aroused from sleep as if smothering; sits up in bed with flushed face, anxious look and rapid hard breathing.' "Burning sensations, which ascend into the chest." "Ebullitions of blood in the chest, after the slightest effort and the least movement, with obstructed respiration, anguish, nausea and weakness, which induces syncope." "Pains and anxiety in the region of the heart." "Pulse hard and quick.' "Palpitation violent with pain; gasping respiration; suddenly awakened after midnight."

Spongia is useful in hypertrophy, angina pectoris, exophthalmic goitre and aneurism.

As with Iodide there is aggravation by heat and amelioration from cold. The time of aggravation is after midnight, especially from 1 to 2 a.m.

Spongia is specially suited to individuals with light hair, fair complexion and lax fibre-the opposite of its congener Iodine.

SULPHUR.

Sulphur causes great irregularity in the distribution of the circulation, flushings and local congestions. It acts predominantly on the venous system and the portal system. It causes a sensation as if the heart were too full, and also the opposite sensation, a feeling or emptiness. Sulphur is a left side medicine and produces more pains in the left side of the chest than the right. "Painful obstruction in left side of chest with anguish and inability to lie on the side affected.'

"Heaviness, fullness and pressure as from a stone on the chest and sternum, principally in the morning, also when coughing, sneezing and yawning." "Pulsations in the chest and sternum."

"Weakness of the chest." "Shooting in the chest or sternum, or extending to the back, or into the left side, principally when coughing, taking a full inspiration, or lifting the arms." "Sensation of coldness or burning in the chest, sometimes extending to the face." "Shootings and blows in region of the heart." "Violent congestion of blood towards the chest and heart, sometimes with ebullitions in the chest uneasiness, faintness, and trembling of the arms." "Sensation of emptiness in the cardiac region, or pressure and sensation as if the heart had not room enough." "Frequent palpitation, sometimes even visible, and with anxiety, principally when going up an ascent.'

These are the local symptoms. The systemic symptoms of Sulphur are well known. It is the "King of antipsoric remedies," with the "sinking sensation" so prominent in psoric patients, well marked and occurring characteristically in the fore-noon from 10 to 12. The typical subject of Sulphur is lean, stoop shouldered, either sanguine or dark, not always very clearly since there is a marked intolerance of water in the Sulphur conditions. Water aggravates all symptoms. Tendency to itching eruptions and an unpleasant body odour.

Warmth aggravates all symptoms, which are worse at night and in the morning. Consequently the sleep is bad; and yet there is great drowsiness in the daytime. Many headaches, full and heavy head, frontal and occipital, with great heat of the vertex. Hot head and cold feet. There is also-hot, sweaty hands and feet; or burning feet, the patient in vain tries to find a cool place for them at night. Acidity. Eructation of mouthfuls of food, very acid, sometime after it has been taken. Constipation, haemorrhoids. In the mental sphere there are-"Melancholy and sadness; uneasiness respecting his condition and prospects; about business affairs so as to become exceedingly unhappy, disgusted with life and despairing of salvation.' "Strong tendency to religious and philosophical reveries with fixed ideas." "Fits of anguish; timidity, and great tendency to be frightened." "Irritability." "Indecision." "Great weakness of memory especially for proper names." A history of suppressed eruptions or discharges is a strong indication for Sulphur.

In the case of a gentleman who suffered from a greatly hypertrophied heart, the result of indulgence in alcohol, occasional doses of Sulphur 1m, F.C., produced a wonderful change for the better. There was a history of previous kidney disease, and when he came under my care he could not bear any exertion, and was unable to lie down in bed at night.

He had fits of breathlessness from exertion or worry. He had a sinking sensation at the pit of the stomach at 11 a.m. and 4 and 7 p.m. It was also brought on when he was in a hot room. A hot room aggravated all his symptoms. He was very nervous and his sleep was bad.

His family doctor told him he might get over Christmas (it was then near the end of November, 1893), but he would not live longer than that. Under Sulphur, chiefly, he became vastly improved in health, and, in addition, he lost all desire for drink.

Sulphur is in close relation to Aconite, Nux vom. Pulsatilla and Psorinum.
TABACUM.
"Palpitation of the heart when lying on left side, better from turning on right side; in attacks at night with tightness of the chest." "Sudden precordial anguish." "Angina pectoris; pallor; features drawn; cannot speak or walk; coldness all over; sudden precordial

anxiety; violent constriction in throat." "Dilated heart; frequent pallor; lividity of face; muscae volitantes; tinnitus aurium; dry cough." "Pulse : quick, full, large; small intermittent; exceedingly slow; soft, full, feeble; feeble and irregular; imperceptible." The mental symptoms of Tabacum are: "Melancholy." "Anguish and inquietude, generally in afternoon, better by weeping."

"Restlessness which prompts continual change of place."

Faintness and nausea are additional indications for Tabacum.

THYROIDIN.

This medicine and its sphere I have so fully dealt with already that I merely mention it in its place here.

VANADIUM.

In his Fifty Reasons for Being a Homoeopath (Reason the Seventh), Dr. Burnett gives a case of neuralgia corresponding to the course of the basilar artery, which he cured with an ammonium salt of Vanadium. There was fatty disease of the liver and atheroma of the arteries, and Dr. Burnett was led to give the medicine on these indications. Vanadium is found most abundantly in lead ores in combination with that metal, which it resembles in producing degeneration of the arterial walls.

VERATRUM ALBUM.

"Violent palpitation of the heart which pushes out the ribs, with choking and severe fits of anxiety." "Palpitation: in the anaemic; nervous; agony of death, legs cold, difficult breathing; better from rest or lying down; with anxiety, and rapid, audible respiration, at night; with prostration of fainting, driving the patient out of bed."

"Angina pectoris; periodical attacks of pain in left chest, or cutting with excessive agony extending to shoulders; general prostration, skin cold and clammy; difficulty of breathing; suffocating constriction of chest, so distressing that he sweats from agony; cramp in limbs." "Pulse: frequent, small, hard; slow, soft, intermittent; very small, irregular; imperceptible."

Cold clammy sweat on forehead indicates Veratrum. "Amorous and religious mania." In rheumatic and other fevers there is delirium with constant talking; "wants to kiss everybody." "Mania, desire to cut and tear everything." "Violent outbreaks, desire to strike." "Great fearfulness; easily frightened; fainting after a fright; consequences of injured pride or honour."

VERATRUM VIRIDE.

"Heart's beat: loud, strong, with great arterial excitement." "Burning, pricking, dull aching in cardiac region." With heart inflammations: "Violent fever; full, hard, bounding pulse; congestion in head without delirium; constant burning pain with oppression of the chest." "Faintness with blindness; when rising from lying; from sudden motions; when lying quietly." "Dreams of water.".

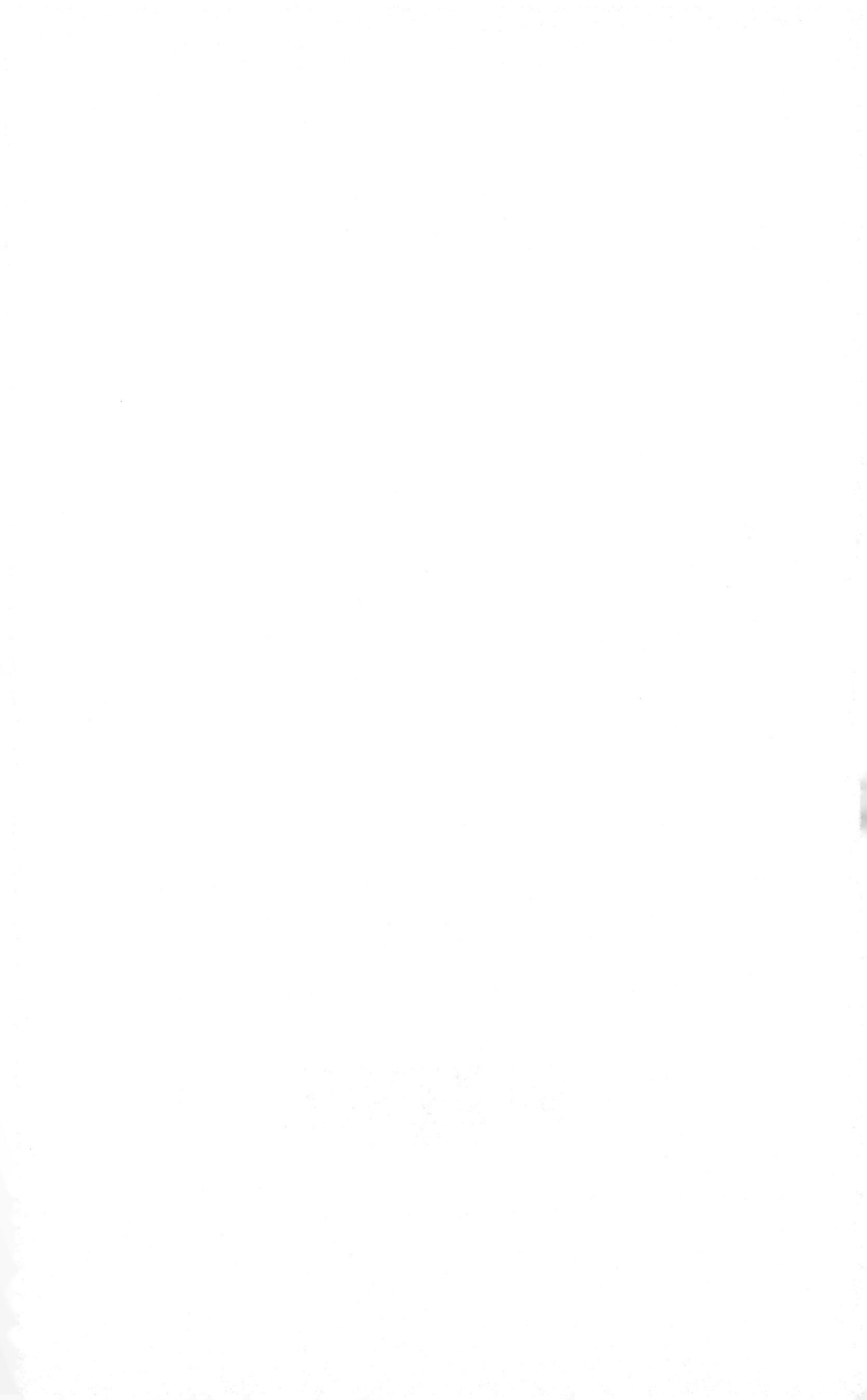

Made in the USA
Monee, IL
04 June 2024